Advances in Celiac Disease

Advances in Celiac Disease

Editor

Luis Rodrigo

MDPI • Basel • Beijing • Wuhan • Barcelona • Belgrade • Manchester • Tokyo • Cluj • Tianjin

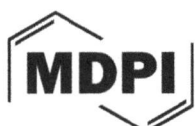

Editor
Luis Rodrigo
Hospital Universitario Central de Asturias (HUCA)
Spain

Editorial Office
MDPI
St. Alban-Anlage 66
4052 Basel, Switzerland

This is a reprint of articles from the Special Issue published online in the open access journal *Medicina* (ISSN 1010-660X) (available at: https://www.mdpi.com/journal/medicina/special_issues/advances_in_celiac_disease).

For citation purposes, cite each article independently as indicated on the article page online and as indicated below:

LastName, A.A.; LastName, B.B.; LastName, C.C. Article Title. *Journal Name* **Year**, *Article Number*, Page Range.

ISBN 978-3-03943-384-1 (Pbk)
ISBN 978-3-03943-385-8 (PDF)

© 2020 by the authors. Articles in this book are Open Access and distributed under the Creative Commons Attribution (CC BY) license, which allows users to download, copy and build upon published articles, as long as the author and publisher are properly credited, which ensures maximum dissemination and a wider impact of our publications.

The book as a whole is distributed by MDPI under the terms and conditions of the Creative Commons license CC BY-NC-ND.

Contents

About the Editor vii

Luis Rodrigo
Celiac Disease: A Common Unrecognized Health Problem with a Very Delayed Diagnosis
Reprinted from: *Medicina* **2020**, *56*, 9, doi:10.3390/medicina56010009 1

Jesús Gilberto Arámburo-Gálvez, Itallo Carvalho Gomes, Tatiane Geralda André, Carlos Eduardo Beltrán-Cárdenas, María Auxiliadora Macêdo-Callou, Élida Mara Braga Rocha, Elaine Aparecida Mye-Takamatu-Watanabe, Vivian Rahmeier-Fietz, Oscar Gerardo Figueroa-Salcido, Feliznando Isidro Cárdenas-Torres, Noé Ontiveros and Francisco Cabrera-Chávez
Translation, Cultural Adaptation, and Evaluation of a Brazilian Portuguese Questionnaire to Estimate the Self-Reported Prevalence of Gluten-Related Disorders and Adherence to Gluten-Free Diet
Reprinted from: *Medicina* **2019**, *55*, 593, doi:10.3390/medicina55090593 5

Tsvetelina Velikova, Martin Shahid, Ekaterina Ivanova-Todorova, Kossara Drenovska, Kalina Tumangelova-Yuzeir, Iskra Altankova and Snejina Vassileva
Celiac-Related Autoantibodies and IL-17A in Bulgarian Patients with Dermatitis Herpetiformis: A Cross-Sectional Study
Reprinted from: *Medicina* **2019**, *55*, 136, doi:10.3390/medicina55050136 15

Ludovico Abenavoli, Stefano Dastoli, Luigi Bennardo, Luigi Boccuto, Maria Passante, Martina Silvestri, Ilaria Proietti, Concetta Potenza, Francesco Luzza and Steven Paul Nisticò
The Skin in Celiac Disease Patients: The Other Side of the Coin
Reprinted from: *Medicina* **2019**, *55*, 578, doi:10.3390/medicina55090578 25

Daniel Vasile Balaban, Alina Popp, Florentina Ionita Radu and Mariana Jinga
Hematologic Manifestations in Celiac Disease—A Practical Review
Reprinted from: *Medicina* **2019**, *55*, 373, doi:10.3390/medicina55070373 43

Mariangela Rondanelli, Milena A. Faliva, Clara Gasparri, Gabriella Peroni, Maurizio Naso, Giulia Picciotto, Antonella Riva, Mara Nichetti, Vittoria Infantino, Tariq A. Alalwan and Simone Perna
Micronutrients Dietary Supplementation Advices for Celiac Patients on Long-Term Gluten-Free Diet with Good Compliance: A Review
Reprinted from: *Medicina* **2019**, *55*, 337, doi:10.3390/medicina55070337 51

Anna Roszkowska, Marta Pawlicka, Anna Mroczek, Kamil Bałabuszek and Barbara Nieradko-Iwanicka
Non-Celiac Gluten Sensitivity: A Review
Reprinted from: *Medicina* **2019**, *55*, 222, doi:10.3390/medicina55060222 69

Cristina Capittini, Annalisa De Silvestri, Chiara Rebuffi, Carmine Tinelli and Dimitri Poddighe
Relevance of HLA-DQB1*02 Allele in the Genetic Predisposition of Children with Celiac Disease: Additional Cues from a Meta-Analysis
Reprinted from: *Medicina* **2019**, *55*, 190, doi:10.3390/medicina55050190 89

Oscar Gerardo Figueroa-Salcido, Noé Ontiveros and Francisco Cabrera-Chavez
Gluten Vehicle and Placebo for Non-Celiac Gluten Sensitivity Assessment
Reprinted from: *Medicina* **2019**, *55*, 117, doi:10.3390/medicina55050117 101

Dimitri Poddighe, Marzhan Rakhimzhanova, Yelena Marchenko and Carlo Catassi
Pediatric Celiac Disease in Central and East Asia: Current Knowledge and Prevalence
Reprinted from: *Medicina* **2019**, *55*, 11, doi:10.3390/medicina55010011 . . . . **111**

About the Editor

Luis Rodrigo, MD is Emeritus Professor of Medicine at the University of Oviedo (Spain). He obtained his PhD in 1975 and has since developed a long teaching and research career spanning 42 years. He has published a total of 695 scientific papers, 413 written in English and the rest in Spanish. He has been the main investigator of a total of 45 clinical trials and has directed 40 doctoral theses. He has written 42 chapters published in books on various topics and is editor of 32 books within his specialty and on related processes. These areas of interest are mainly related to celiac disease and autoimmune-associated diseases, *Helicobacter pylori*, chronic HCV infections, and all types of infectious diseases generally. His research output is represented by a h-index of 49.

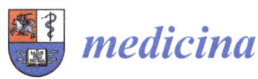

Editorial

Celiac Disease: A Common Unrecognized Health Problem with a Very Delayed Diagnosis

Luis Rodrigo

Gastroenterology Unit, Hospital Universitario Central de Asturias, 33011 Oviedo, Asturias, Spain; lrodrigosaez@gmail.com

Received: 18 December 2019; Accepted: 23 December 2019; Published: 26 December 2019

Celiac disease (CD) is a clinical entity of autoimmune nature, related to the presence of a permanent gluten intolerance that affects genetically predisposed individuals, producing a chronic inflammation process that usually occurs in the small bowel. It is accompanied by a relatively high frequency of simultaneous or successive involvement of various extra-digestive organs over time [1].

CD has an extensive epidemiological distribution, affecting all countries and ethnicities. Its average prevalence is 1–2% in the general population, with slight variations between geographical areas. It can arise at any time during the life-course, but predominantly appears in middle age, and up to 20% of cases are diagnosed in patients older than 60 years. It is also clearly predominant in women (average ratio 2:1, female:male) [2,3].

Clinical manifestations vary considerably in relation to the age of presentation and to various associated exogenous factors. In children, it usually begins to manifest itself in conjunction with the introduction into their diet of foodstuffs containing wheat flour (e.g., porridge) from six months of age. In the most severe cases, the clinical symptoms appear before the age of two years. In general, digestive symptoms predominate, such as chronic diarrhea, bloating and weight loss, the "classic triad" of symptoms, and are not necessarily accompanied by a malabsorption syndrome. Other accompanying symptoms are anorexia, vomiting, reflux and accentuated irritability, along with episodes of constipation that can be frequent and prolonged [4,5].

When the disease appears in older children or adolescents, several extraintestinal manifestations, such as headaches, arthritis, anemia and accentuated asthenia, among others, may appear in addition to digestive symptoms [6].

The forms of CD presentation are very varied in adults, with frequent associations of intestinal and extradigestive symptoms, often referred to as "atypical forms". Among them are serious conditions, such as chronic anemia, osteoporosis, a variety of skin lesions, polyneuritis, migraines, persistent liver test abnormalities, dysmenorrhea, amenorrhea, fertility disorders, recurrent abortions and mood changes (e.g., irritability and depression). Dermatitis herpetiformis is the skin lesion most frequently associated with CD, appearing in up to 25% of cases. It is easily recognized and highly suspicious. Gluten is the agent mainly responsible for the condition, and its withdrawal is definitively the most effective treatment.

Initial clinical screening most often involves determining levels of serological markers, which are circulating antibodies directed against some compound of gluten proteins, sensitivity or the enzymes that metabolize it. The most commonly used are class 2 anti-tissue transglutaminase antibodies, which are close to 90% efficacious in cases with intestinal villus atrophy. However, their diagnostic sensitivity is remarkably low, at 30–40%, for cases without villous atrophy, so that one or more negative determinations does not in any way rule out the possibility that an established CD is present [7].

There are two known genetic markers, both belonging to the HLA-II class, available for routine clinical use in the study of patients with CD. HLA-DQ2 is the most frequent, being positive in 90% of celiac patients, while HLA-DQ8 is much less common (5–8%). The two genetic markers are simultaneously negative in a small percentage of patients (<2–3%). The presence of both genetic markers is considered to be a necessary, but not sufficient condition for the diagnosis, as they also occur in up to 30% of the general non-celiac population.

The spectrum of duodenal histological changes in CD has expanded greatly since the inclusion of the new criteria introduced by Marsh in 1992 [8]. He successfully included celiac patients without villous atrophy, classifying them as type 1 when there was only an increased intraepithelial lymphocytosis (LIES) (>25% of LIES, per 100 epithelial cells). Type 2 is characterized by the presence of crypt hyperplasia without atrophy. Type 3, showing villous atrophy, is subdivided into three categories: mild (3a), moderate (3b) and intense (3c). Other classifications have since appeared, but they are basically very similar to the original Marsh classification [9,10].

The most important step towards achieving a diagnosis of CD is that every doctor looks for this entity and includes it in their differential process before a series of symptoms, and not only digestive but also long-term extra-intestinal usually. This is not achieved solely on the basis of clinical data and exploratory findings, but aided by analytical alterations, serological data, genetic markers and duodenal histopathological findings. If, after this process, reasonable doubts remain about its presence, it may be tentatively proposed that the patient follows a gluten-free diet (GFD) for at least six months, to assess their degree of response. Although a GFD is the only available and effective treatment, it should be made clear that it must be followed strictly and maintained for the rest of the patient's life, avoiding transgressions and contamination [11].

Diagnosis is often delayed, the time following symptom onset being highly variable in adults, sometimes taking as long as 12 years. Barriers to accurate and timely diagnosis include atypical presentation, physicians' lack of awareness about current diagnostic criteria, misdiagnosis and general practitioners' limited access to specialists [12]. In a survey of 611 CD patients in Finland, 332 (54%) reported a delay in diagnosis of more than three years. This delay predisposed patients to reduced well-being and increased recourse to medicines and health care services, before the diagnosis and one year after diagnosis [13]. New guidelines have been issued for children who exhibit high serum TGT titers of more than ten times the normal value. In such cases it is not considered necessary to perform duodenal biopsies to confirm the diagnosis [14].

Conflicts of Interest: The author declares no conflict of interest.

References

1. Ludvigsson, J.F.; Bai, J.C.; Biagi, F.; Card, T.R.; Ciacci, C.; Ciclitira, P.J.; Green, P.H.; Hadjivassiliou, M.; Holdoway, A.; van Heel, D.A.; et al. Diagnosis and management of adult coeliac disease: Guidelines from the British Society of Gastroenterology. *Gut* **2014**, *63*, 1210–1228. [CrossRef] [PubMed]
2. Kang, J.Y.; Kang, A.H.; Green, A.; Gwee, K.A.; Ho, K.Y. Systematic review: Worldwide variation in the frequency of coeliac disease and changes over time. *Aliment. Pharmacol. Ther.* **2013**, *38*, 226–245. [CrossRef] [PubMed]
3. Vaquero, L.; Caminero, A.; Nuñez, A.; Hernando, M.; Iglesias, C.; Casqueiro, J.; Vivas, S. Coeliac disease screening in first-degree relatives on the basis of biopsy and genetic risk. *Eur. J. Gastroenterol. Hepatol.* **2014**, *26*, 263–267. [CrossRef] [PubMed]
4. Volta, U.; Caio, G.; Stanghellini, V.; De Giorgio, R. The changing clinical profile of celiac disease: A 15-year experience (1998–2012) in an Italian referral center. *BMC Gastroenterol.* **2014**, *14*, 194. [CrossRef] [PubMed]
5. Vivas, S.; Ruiz de Morales, J.M.; Fernandez, M.; Hernando, M.; Herrero, B.; Casqueiro, J.; Gutierrez, S. Age-related clinical, serological, and histopathological features of celiac disease. *Am. J. Gastroenterol.* **2008**, *103*, 2360–2365. [CrossRef] [PubMed]
6. Lionetti, E.; Catassi, C. New clues in celiac disease epidemiology, pathogenesis, clinical manifestations, and treatment. *Int. Rev. Immunol.* **2011**, *30*, 219–231. [CrossRef] [PubMed]
7. Bonaci-Nikolic, B.; Andrejevic, S.; Radlovic, N.; Davidovic, I.; Sofronic, L.; Spuran, M.; Micev, M.; Nikolic, M.M. Serological and clinical comparison of children and adults with anti-endomysial antibodies. *J. Clin. Immunol.* **2007**, *27*, 163–171. [CrossRef] [PubMed]

8. Marsh, M.N. Gluten, major histocompatibility complex, and the small intestine A molecular and immunobiologic approach to the spectrum of gluten sensitivity ('celiac sprue'). *Gastroenterology* **1992**, *102*, 330–354. [CrossRef]
9. Lauret, E.; Rodrigo, L. Celiac disease and autoimmune-associated conditions. *BioMed Res. Int.* **2013**, *2013*, 127589. [CrossRef] [PubMed]
10. Santolaria Piedrafita, S.; Fernández Bañares, F. Gluten-sensitive enteropathy and functional dyspepsia. *Gastroenterol. Hepatol.* **2012**, *35*, 78–88. [CrossRef] [PubMed]
11. Sainsbury, A.; Sanders, D.S.; Ford, A.C. Prevalence of irritable bowel syndrome-type symptoms in patients with celiac disease: A meta-analysis. *Clin. Gastroenterol. Hepatol.* **2013**, *11*, 359–365. [CrossRef] [PubMed]
12. Cichewicz, A.B.; Mearns, E.S.; Taylor, A.; Boulanger, T.; Gerber, M.; Leffler, D.A.; Drahos, J.; Sanders, D.S.; Thomas Craig, K.J.; Lebwohl, B. Diagnosis and treatment patterns in celiac disease. *Dig. Dis. Sci.* **2019**, *64*, 2095–2106. [CrossRef]
13. Fuchs, V.; Kurppa, K.; Huhtala, H.; Mäki, M.; Kekkonen, L.; Kaukinen, K. Delayed celiac disease diagnosis predisposes to reduced quality of life and incremental use of health care services and medicines: A prospective nationwide study. *United Eur. Gastroenterol. J.* **2018**, *6*, 567–575. [CrossRef]
14. Husby, S.; Koletzko, S.; Korponay-Szabó, I.R.; Mearin, M.L.; Phillips, A.; Shamir, R.; Troncone, R.; Giersiepen, K.; Branski, D.; Catassi, C.; et al. European Society for Pediatric Gastroenterology, Hepatology, and Nutrition guidelines for the diagnosis of coeliac disease. *J. Pediatr. Gastroenterol. Nutr.* **2012**, *54*, 136–160. [CrossRef] [PubMed]

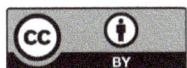

© 2019 by the author. Licensee MDPI, Basel, Switzerland. This article is an open access article distributed under the terms and conditions of the Creative Commons Attribution (CC BY) license (http://creativecommons.org/licenses/by/4.0/).

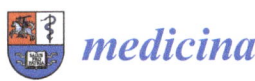

Article

Translation, Cultural Adaptation, and Evaluation of a Brazilian Portuguese Questionnaire to Estimate the Self-Reported Prevalence of Gluten-Related Disorders and Adherence to Gluten-Free Diet

Jesús Gilberto Arámburo-Gálvez [1,2], Itallo Carvalho Gomes [3], Tatiane Geralda André [3], Carlos Eduardo Beltrán-Cárdenas [1], María Auxiliadora Macêdo-Callou [4], Élida Mara Braga Rocha [4], Elaine Aparecida Mye-Takamatu-Watanabe [5], Vivian Rahmeier-Fietz [5], Oscar Gerardo Figueroa-Salcido [1,2], Feliznando Isidro Cárdenas-Torres [1], Noé Ontiveros [6,*] and Francisco Cabrera-Chávez [1,*]

1. Unidad Academica de Ciencias de la Nutrición y Gastronomia, Universidad Autónoma de Sinaloa, Culiacán, Sinaloa 80019, Mexico; gilberto.aramburo.g@gmail.com (J.G.A.-G.); carlos.1.beltran@hotmail.com (C.E.B.-C.); gerardofs95@hotmail.com (O.G.F.-S.); feliznandoc@hotmail.com (F.I.C.-T.)
2. Posgrado en Ciencias de la Salud, División de Ciencias Biológicas y de la Salud, Universidad de Sonora, Hermosillo, Sonora 83000, Mexico
3. Programa de Maestría en Ciencias en Enfermeria, Facultad de Enfermería, Los Mochis, Sinaloa 81220, Mexico; carvalhoitallo@gmail.com (I.C.G.); tatianegrandre@gmail.com (T.G.A.)
4. Faculdade de Juazeiro do Norte, Juazeiro do Norte, Ceará 63010-215, Brazil; auxiliadora.callou@fjn.edu.br (M.A.M.-C.); elidamara@usp.br (É.M.B.R.)
5. Universidade Estadual de Mato Grosso do Sul, Dourados, Mato Grosso do Sul 79804-970, Brazil; swatanab@terra.com.br (E.A.M.-T.-W.); vivian@uems.br (V.R.-F.)
6. Division of Sciences and Engineering, Department of Chemical, Biological, and Agricultural Sciences (DC-QB), Clinical and Research Laboratory (LACIUS, URS), University of Sonora, Navojoa 85880, Sonora, Mexico
* Correspondence: noe.ontiveros@unison.mx (N.O.); fcabrera@uas.edu.mx (F.C.-C.)

Received: 28 June 2019; Accepted: 11 September 2019; Published: 15 September 2019

Abstract: *Background*: A Spanish version of a questionnaire intended to estimate, at the population level, the prevalence rates of self-reported gluten-related disorders and adherence to gluten-free diets has been applied in four Latin American countries. However, idiom issues have hampered the questionnaire application in the Brazilian population. Thus, the aim of the present study was to carry out a translation, cultural adaptation, and evaluation of a Brazilian Portuguese questionnaire to estimate the self-reported prevalence of gluten-related disorders and adherence to gluten-free diets in a Brazilian population. *Materials and Methods*: Two bilingual Portuguese–Spanish health professionals carried out the translation of the original Spanish version of the questionnaire to Brazilian-Portuguese. Matching between the two translations was evaluated using the WCopyFind.4.1.5 software. Words in conflict were conciliated, and the conciliated version of the Brazilian Portuguese instrument was evaluated to determine its clarity, comprehension, and consistency. A pilot study was carried out using an online platform. *Results*: The two questionnaires translated into Brazilian Portuguese were highly matched (81.8%–84.1%). The questions of the conciliated questionnaire were clear and comprehensible with a high agreement among the evaluators ($n = 64$) (average Kendall's W score was 0.875). The participants did not suggest re-wording of questions. The answers to the questions were consistent after two applications of the questionnaire (Cohen's k = 0.869). The pilot online survey yielded low response rates (9.0%) highlighting the need for face-to-face interviews. *Conclusions*: The translation and evaluation of a Brazilian Portuguese questionnaire to estimate the self-reported prevalence rates of gluten-related disorders and adherence to gluten-free diets was carried out. The instrument is clear, comprehensible, and generates reproducible results in the target population. Further survey studies involving face-to-face interviews are warranted.

Keywords: celiac disease; gluten-free diet; gluten-related disorders; NCGS; self-report; survey studies

1. Introduction

The spectrum of gluten-related disorders (GRD) involves celiac disease (CD), wheat allergy and non-celiac gluten sensitivity (NCGS). Patients under this spectrum should follow a gluten-free diet (GFD) to avoid the gastrointestinal and/or extraintestinal symptoms triggered by gluten. In fact, survey studies have proven that following a GFD can improve the health-related quality of life in CD patients in spite of the difficulties of following the diet [1]. Different from wheat allergy and NCGS, untreated CD could affect the nutritional status and predispose to other conditions such as osteoporosis [2,3], anemia [4], and intestinal T-cell lymphoma [5]. On its own, following a GFD without medical/dietitian advice can predispose not only to deficiencies in micronutrients, but also to low fiber intake [6,7] increasing the risk of dyslipidemia [8,9]. Notably, recent survey-based studies carried out in Latin American countries have shown that both CD and NCGS are largely underdiagnosed in Mexico, Colombia, and El Salvador, and that most people following a GFD are doing it for reasons other than health related benefits, as well as without medical advice [10–12]. This is not the case in Argentina, a country that has implemented programs for the detection of CD and for ameliorating the economic burden of following a GFD [13]. The questionnaire utilized in these studies is a Spanish version, and this has hampered its application in the Brazilian population. Recently, an Italian instrument [14] designed to estimate the prevalence of NCGS in clinical settings has been translated to Brazilian Portuguese [15], but a validated questionnaire intended to evaluate, at population level, the self-reported prevalence of GRD and adherence to a GFD in Brazilians is not available yet. Thus, as part of an attempt to expose the magnitude and relevance of the underdiagnosis of GRD and the adherence to GFD in the Latin American region, the aim of the present work is to generate and test a Brazilian Portuguese version of a validated Spanish questionnaire designed to estimate the self-reported prevalence of GRD and adherence to a GFD.

2. Materials and Methods

2.1. Questionnaire

The questionnaire is based on a previously designed and tested instrument that is utilized in Spanish-speaking populations [10–13]. The questionnaire includes 2 sections. The first section was designed for those who report adverse reactions after wheat/gluten ingestion, and the second one for those who do not report them. The participants should answer questions related to the symptoms triggered after gluten ingestion, time of appearance of the symptoms, adherence to a GFD or gluten avoidance and the motivations of doing so, among other questions (Supplementary Material Section S1).

2.2. Translation and Back-Translation

The translation process of the questionnaire was carried out as previously described, with minor changes [16,17]. The procedure was as follows: two health professionals, Portuguese–Spanish bilingual, but also Brazilian Portuguese native speakers, realized the translation of the questionnaire from Spanish to Brazilian Portuguese (TBP1 and TBP2). The matches between translations were analyzed using the WCopyFind.4.1.5 software (Charlottesville, VA, USA) to determine literal match by words (ignoring phrases, all punctuations, outer punctuations, numbers, letter case, and skipping non-words, selecting Brazilian-Portuguese as the base language). After conciliation of the words in conflict (words that did not match) by the Spanish-Portuguese translators, a conciliate version of the questionnaire was elaborated and back-translated to Spanish by two Spanish-Portuguese bilingual professionals who were also Spanish native speakers. The match between the back-translated questionnaires (from Brazilian Portuguese to Spanish; two versions) and the match between each back-translated version with the original Spanish version of the questionnaire were evaluated as previously described (selecting Mexican Spanish as the base language). All matches were reported as percentage.

2.3. Questionnaire Clarity, Comprehension and Wording of Questions Evaluation

Clarity and comprehension of the conciliated questionnaire in Brazilian Portuguese was evaluated as previously described [10,16]. A digital version of the Brazilian Portuguese questionnaire was constructed using the SurveyMonkey platform (San Mateo, CA, USA). Brazilian Portuguese native speakers ($n = 64$) received a text message with the link to the questionnaire. Afterwards, participants proceeded to evaluate the clarity and comprehension of all the questions.

The evaluation was initially performed using a numerical scale from 0 to 10 (0 = very easy to understand; 10 = very difficult to understand). Questions rated with values ≤3 were considered as clear and comprehensible, therefore, rewording was not required [10]. Results were reported with 95% confidence intervals. Furthermore, clarity/comprehension was evaluated using a cognitive survey that evaluated each item/question in a three-point ordinal scale; 1: Clear and comprehensible, 2: Difficult to understand, and 3: Incomprehensible [16]. Agreement among participants was evaluated using the Kendall's W coefficient of concordance, ranging from 0 (no agreement) to 1 (complete agreement). A W value ≥ 0.66 was considered as an adequate agreement among the participants. Additionally, to ensure the comprehension of each question, the participants were to answer the following question: In case you do not understand the question, how would you write it? This option was provided if the participants did not correctly understand some questions, or if they thought that there was a more comprehensible way to write the item.

2.4. Questionnaire Test-Retest Consistency

The questionnaire reproducibility was evaluated in a cohort of subjects who reported adverse reactions to wheat/gluten ($n = 12$), as well as in another cohort who reported adverse reactions to foods other than gluten ($n = 8$). Participants answered the questionnaire twice. The time period interval between the first and second application of the questionnaire was at least one week. The reproducibility of the questionnaire was evaluated with Cohen's k coefficient tests.

2.5. Pilot Survey

After the clarity/comprehension and consistency evaluation process, a digital version of the conciliated Brazilian-Portuguese questionnaire (Supplementary Material Section S2) was sent to 966 Brazilian health sciences students from Faculdade do Juazeiro do Norte in Juazeiro do Norte, Ceará, Brazil using the SurveyMonkey platform (San Mateo, CA, USA). The first page of the survey showed a general description of the project and presented the consent form. All data were collected in June 2019. Inclusion criteria were as follows: subjects must be aged ≥ 18 years old, and able to read and answer the questionnaire by themselves. Exclusion criteria were as follows: subjects being < 18 years old or not being able to complete the questionnaire by themselves. Individuals were classified according to previously published definitions on GRD [12] (Supplementary Material Section S3).

2.6. Statistical Analysis and Ethical Issues

Statistical analysis was carried out using PASW statistics version 25.0 (SPSS Inc., Chicago, IL, USA). Total numbers, percentages, and 95% confidence intervals (CI) were analyzed according to a set of descriptive statistics. A p value < 0.05 was considered as statistically significant. OpenEpi software version 3.03a (Atlanta, GA, USA) was used to estimate the prevalence rates (95% CI) per 100 inhabitants. This study was approved by the Research Ethics Committee of the Faculdade do Juazeiro do norte (Número do Parecer: 3.382.689).

3. Results

3.1. Questionnaire Translation and Back-Translation

The complete flow chart and the results of the evaluation of translation, clarity, comprehensibility, and consistency of the questionnaire are shown in Figure 1. Two native Brazilian Portuguese speakers carried out the translations from Spanish to Brazilian Portuguese. Translations to Brazilian-Portuguese (TBP1 and 2) had more than 80% of an overall match between them (TBP1 matched 81.8% with TBP2 and TBP2 matched 84.1% with TBP1). Most of the items in conflict were synonymous in Brazilian Portuguese with the same meaning in Spanish language. After agreement by the translators, the best synonymous were selected to have a conciliated version of the questionnaire translated to Brazilian Portuguese. The back-translations (two versions) of the conciliated Brazilian Portuguese version of the instrument matched 93.7% and 85.4% with the original Spanish version.

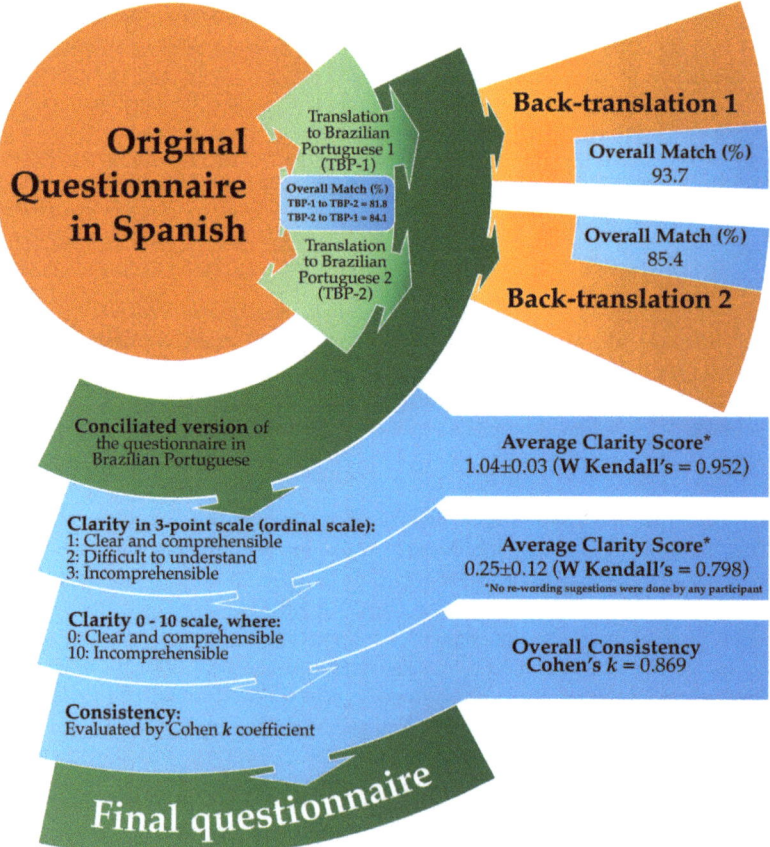

Figure 1. Flow chart of the translation of the questionnaire and the results of the evaluations on matches (between translations 1 and 2 from Spanish to Brazilian Portuguese, and between back-translations to Spanish compared to the original questionnaire), clarity, comprehension, and consistency.

3.2. Questionnaire Clarity/Comprehension

Sixty-four Brazilian Portuguese native speakers (38 females, 26 males; 18–55 years old) evaluated clarity/comprehensibility using a continuous scale (0: clear and comprehensible, 10: incomprehensible).

On the bases of this evaluation, the average of the clarity score was 0.25 (CI, 95%: 0.03–0.53; values ranged from 0 to 9) and the Kendall's W score was 0.798. Using the three-point ordinal scale, the average of the clarity score was 1.04. This value is very close to "clear and comprehensible" and, according to the Kendall's W score obtained (0.952), involves a high concordance among the individuals' answers to the questions. Importantly, when the participants were asked for the questions' re-writing to improve the understanding, neither re-wording nor suggestions for changes were reported.

3.3. Questionnaire Consistency

Twenty participants who reported adverse reactions to gluten or to other foods answered the questionnaire twice (12 females and 8 males). The concordance between the first and the second application of the questionnaire was measured individually, and the average of Cohen's k coefficient was 0.869 (Figure 1). This k value can be interpreted as an almost perfect concordance.

3.4. Pilot Study

A total of 966 health sciences students received the link to answer the questionnaire. The response rate was 9.0% ($n = 87$), but 13 subjects had to be excluded due to their proportioned incomplete demographic data or responses. Thus, a total of 74 valid questionnaires were considered for prevalence estimations. The proportion of male/female was 24.3%: 75.6% (male: 18; female: 56). Average age was 25 ± 6.6 years. The most commonly self-reported, physician-diagnosed conditions were psychiatric diseases (9.45%; IC 95%), irritable bowel syndrome (8.1%; IC 95% 3.88–18.52), diabetes, lactose intolerance, and allergies (6.75%; IC 2.23–15.07, each). However, due to the reduced number of participants, risk analysis between Self-Reported Gluten Sensitivity (SR-GS) and non-Self-Reported Gluten Sensitivity (non-SR-GS) conditions could not be calculated.

Prevalence rates estimations of GRD and other adverse foods reactions are shown in the Table 1. Adverse reactions to wheat/gluten were reported by 16.21% of the participants, though, only two fulfilled criteria for SR-GS (2.70%) (Supplementary Material Section S3). The prevalence rates of wheat allergy and NCGS were 1.35% each. No male fulfilled the criteria for either wheat allergy or NCGS. Physician diagnosis of CD was not reported in this pilot study. The prevalence rate of adherence to a GFD was higher in females than in males, while the prevalence rate of wheat/gluten avoiders was slightly higher in males than in females ($p > 0.05$).

The characteristics of the individuals following a GFD are shown in Figure 2. It should be noted that almost all participants who were following a GFD (75%) and those that were avoiding wheat/gluten containing foods (75%) fulfilled criteria for non-SR-GS. Regarding the motivations for following a GFD, in the non-SR-GS group the most frequent motivation was weight control (50%), while in the SR-GS group was the symptomatic relapse. Similar results were obtained in the wheat/gluten avoiders group. All participants who were following a GFD reported to be under the supervision of a dietitian to follow the diet. Ten individuals reported recurrent gastrointestinal and/or extra-intestinal symptoms triggered after the ingestion of wheat/gluten containing foods. Bloating (80%), abdominal pain (80%), nausea (60%), stomachache (60%), and reflux (60%) were the most commonly reported gastrointestinal symptoms. On the other hand, lack of wellbeing (60%), tiredness (40%), and muscular pain (40%) were the most commonly reported extra-intestinal symptoms.

Table 1. Self-reported prevalence rates.

Assessment	(+) Cases	Mean Age in Years (Range)	Prevalence by Gender (95% CI)	p-Value	General Prevalence (95% CI)
Adverse reaction to foods	n = 24 M = 6 F = 18	27 (19–47)	M = 33.33 (13.34–59.01) F = 32.14 (20.28–45.96)	0.999	32.43 (22.0–44.32)
Adverse reaction to wheat/gluten	n = 12 M = 3 F = 9	30 (20–47)	M = 16.66 (3.57–41.42) F = 16.07 (7.62–28.33)	0.999	16.21 (8.67–26.61)
Self-Reported Gluten sensitivity (SR-GS)	n = 2 M = 0 F = 2	27 (20–34)	M = 0 (0.0–18.53) F = 3.57 (0.43–12.31)	0.999	2.70 (0.32–9.42)
SR-PD Celiac disease	n = 0	—	—	—	—
Wheat allergy	n = 1 M = 0 F = 1	20 (N/D)	M = 0 (0.0–18.53) F = 1.29 (0.22–6.99)	0.999	1.35 (0.03–7.30)
NCGS	n = 1 M = 0 F = 1	34 (N/D)	M = 0 (0.0–18.53) F = 1.29 (0.22–6.99)	0.999	1.35 (0.03–7.30)
Adherence to GFD	n = 8 M = 1 F = 7	25 (20–41)	M = 1.29 (0.22–6.99) F = 9.09 (4.47–17.6)	0.671	10.81 (4.78–20.19)
Avoid wheat/gluten-containing foods	n = 12 M = 3 F = 9	26 (20–41)	M = 16.66 (3.57–41.42) F = 16.07 (7.62–28.33)	0.999	16.21 (8.67–26.61)

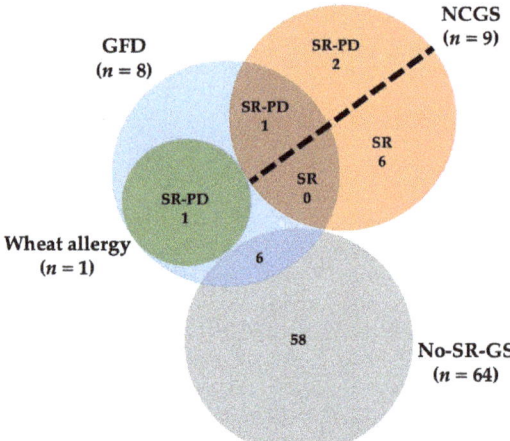

Figure 2. Characteristics of the participants who were following a GFD. SR-PD: Self-reported Physician-Diagnosed; SR: Self-reported; GFD: Gluten-free Diet; NCGS: Non-Celiac Gluten Sensitivity; Non-SR-GS: Non-self-reported Gluten Sensitivity.

4. Discussion

Survey-based studies are useful to estimate the prevalence rates of several conditions and set the ground for further epidemiological studies based on objective diagnostic criteria. The results of survey studies can be interpreted in different ways. Particular attention needed to be given to the most underdiagnosed conditions and those conditions for which there is a lack of sensitive and specific biomarkers, such as CD and NCGS, respectively. In this context, a questionnaire intended to evaluate the self-reported prevalence of GRD and the adherence to a GFD in Spanish-speaking populations was applied in four Latin American countries [10–13]. However, idiom issues hampered the application of this instrument in Brazilian Portuguese speakers, the largest population in South America. To fill this gap, the questionnaire was translated to Brazilian Portuguese and systematically tested. The translations of the questionnaire from Spanish to Brazilian Portuguese matched in high percentage and most of the items in conflict were words with the same meaning. The similarity between Spanish and Portuguese is the highest among romance languages [18], thus allowing for the facilitation of the translation of the questionnaire and, at the same time, it could improve the matching among the translations carried out by different translators. Back-translation is a process necessary to verify the accuracy of the original translation [19] and to reduce any discrepancies between the original version of the instrument and the back-translated version [20]. The overall matching between the back-translated versions with the original Spanish version indicates a high similarity between them. This supports the notion that the conciliated version of the questionnaire in Brazilian-Portuguese mirrors the original Spanish version.

Precision evaluation of the words utilized in a questionnaire is essential to avoid misinterpretation or incomprehension of the formulated questions [21]. In the present study, the outcome of the clarity/comprehension evaluation using a continuous scale was excellent (0.25; where 0 means clear and comprehensible). This indicated that the conciliated version of the questionnaire in Brazilian Portuguese language was clear and comprehensible. Importantly, the participants did not suggest re-writing of questions. These results are similar to those reported in the clarity/comprehension evaluation of the original Spanish version of the questionnaire [10]. To corroborate the clarity/comprehension data obtained in the present study, additional tests based on a three-point ordinal scale were carried out. The results of these tests corroborate that the Brazilian-Portuguese version of the questionnaire was clear and comprehensible. Additionally, the average of the Kendall's W coefficient for the clarity/comprehension evaluation highlighted a very high agreement among the evaluations of the participants [22].

The consistency in the answers to each question of the questionnaire by the same individual was also evaluated. The questionnaire was applied twice at different moments, allowing at least one-week intervals to pass between the two applications. The consistency evaluated as the k coefficient value was 0.869, which can be considered an excellent agreement between the two applications of the questionnaire [23]. This result is similar to that reported for the original Spanish version of the instrument [10].

Online survey studies have gained attention, as the staff requirement to collect data and printing costs can be kept to a minimum. Under these bases, a pilot online survey study was carried out using the instrument generated. However, a very low response rate was reported (9.0%). In line with this, several survey-based studies, conducted using internet platforms, have reported similar and even lower response rates [24]. On the contrary, previous studies have reported high response rates (53.3 to 92.0%) using the Spanish version of the questionnaire utilized in this pilot study, but conducting the survey on the bases of face-to-face interviews in public places instead of using internet platforms [10–13]. The prevalence data generated in the present online pilot survey study should be interpreted with caution, as the response rate was quite low, and the sample was limited to Brazilian health sciences students. The same applies for the data related to the gastrointestinal and extra-intestinal symptoms reported. The main contribution of the online pilot survey study carried out in the present work is that it highlights the need to perform face-to-face interviews to successfully utilize the Brazilian-Portuguese version of the questionnaire intended to evaluate the self-reported prevalence of GRD and adherence to a GFD.

5. Conclusions

In this study, a questionnaire intended to estimate the prevalence of self-reported GRD and adherence to a GFD was translated to Brazilian Portuguese and tested. The questionnaire was clear, comprehensible, and generated reproducible results in the target population. The questionnaire should ideally be applied preferentially on the bases of face-to-face interviews instead of using online platforms. This strategy can help to improve the response rate and minimize bias in order to generate representative results. The present study provides an instrument to estimate the prevalence of self-reported GRD and adherence to a GFD in Brazilian Portuguese native speakers, a community that represents almost half of the South America population.

Supplementary Materials: The following are available online at http://www.mdpi.com/1010-660X/55/9/593/s1, Supplementary Material Section S1: Questionnaire in English; Supplementary Material Section S2: Conciliated version of the questionnaire in Brazilian Portuguese; Supplementary Material Section S3: Definition and criteria of gluten-related disorders.

Author Contributions: Conceptualization, N.O. and F.C.-C.; data curation, J.G.A.-G. and C.E.B.-C.; formal analysis, O.G.F.-S., F.I.C.-T., N.O. and F.C.-C.; investigation, J.G.A.-G., M.A.M.-C., É.M.B.R., E.A.M.-T.-W., V.R.-F., O.G.F.-S., F.I.C.-T., N.O. and F.C.-C.; methodology, J.G.A.-G., I.C.G., T.G.A., C.E.B.-C., M.A.M.-C., É.M.B.R., E.A.M.-T.-W., V.R.-F., O.G.F.-S. and F.I.C.-T.; resources, N.O. and F.C.-C.; visualization, F.I.C.-T., N.O. and F.C.-C.; writing—original draft, J.G.A.-G., N.O. and F.C.-C.; writing—review and editing, I.C.G., T.G.A., C.E.B.-C., M.A.M.-C., É.M.B.R., E.A.M.-T.-W., V.R.-F., O.G.F.-S., F.I.C.-T., N.O. and F.C.-C.

Funding: This research received no external funding.

Acknowledgments: We acknowledge the technical support by Yolanda Irene Aguilar Hinojosa and Jose Pedro Mendes Alves Palmela. We acknowledge the postgraduate fellowships given to I.C.G., T.G.A., and F.I.C.-T., by the Mexican Council for Science and Technology (CONACyT).

Conflicts of Interest: The authors declare no conflict of interest.

References

1. Casellas, F.; Rodrigo, L.; Lucendo, A.J.; Fernández-Bañares, F.; Molina-Infante, J.; Vivas, S.; Rosinach, M.; Dueñas, C.; López-Vivancos, J. Benefit on health-related quality of life of adherence to gluten-free diet in adult patients with celiac disease. *Rev. Española Enferm. Dig.* **2015**, *107*, 196–201.
2. Walker, M.D.; Williams, J.; Lewis, S.K.; Bai, J.C.; Lebwohl, B.; Green, P.H.R. Measurement of forearm bone density by dual energy x-ray absorptiometry increases the prevalence of osteoporosis in men with celiac disease. *Clin. Gastroenterol. Hepatol.* **2019**, 1–8. [CrossRef] [PubMed]
3. Ganji, R.; Moghbeli, M.; Sadeghi, R.; Bayat, G.; Ganji, A. Prevalence of osteoporosis and osteopenia in men and premenopausal women with celiac disease: A systematic review. *Nutr. J.* **2019**, *18*, 9. [CrossRef] [PubMed]
4. Freeman, H.J. Iron deficiency anemia in celiac disease. *World J. Gastroenterol.* **2015**, *21*, 9233–9238. [CrossRef] [PubMed]
5. Malamut, G.; Chandesris, O.; Verkarre, V.; Meresse, B.; Callens, C.; Macintyre, E.; Bouhnik, Y.; Gornet, J.M.; Allez, M.; Jian, R.; et al. Enteropathy associated T cell lymphoma in celiac disease: A large retrospective study. *Dig. Liver Dis.* **2013**, *45*, 377–384. [CrossRef] [PubMed]
6. Wild, D.; Robins, G.G.; Burley, V.J.; Howdle, P.D. Evidence of high sugar intake, and low fibre and mineral intake, in the gluten-free diet. *Aliment. Pharmacol. Ther.* **2010**, *32*, 573–581. [CrossRef]
7. Taetzsch, A.; Das, S.K.; Brown, C.; Krauss, A.; Silver, R.E.; Roberts, S.B. Are gluten-free diets more nutritious? An evaluation of self-selected and recommended gluten-free and gluten-containing dietary patterns. *Nutrients* **2018**, *10*, 1881. [CrossRef]
8. Narayan, S.; Lakshmipriya, N.; Vaidya, R.; Bai, M.R.; Sudha, V.; Krishnaswamy, K.; Unnikrishnan, R.; Anjana, R.M.; Mohan, V. Association of dietary fiber intake with serum total cholesterol and low density lipoprotein cholesterol levels in Urban Asian-Indian adults with type 2 diabetes. *Indian J. Endocrinol. Metab.* **2014**, *18*, 624–630.
9. Zhou, Q.; Wu, J.; Tang, J.; Wang, J.-J.; Lu, C.-H.; Wang, P.-X. Beneficial effect of higher dietary fiber intake on plasma HDL-C and TC/HDL-C ratio among chinese rural-to-urban migrant workers. *Int. J. Environ. Res. Public Health* **2015**, *12*, 4726–4738. [CrossRef]
10. Ontiveros, N.; López-Gallardo, J.A.; Vergara-Jiménez, M.J.; Cabrera-Chávez, F. Self-reported prevalence of symptomatic adverse reactions to gluten and adherence to gluten-free diet in an adult mexican population. *Nutrients* **2015**, *7*, 6000–6015. [CrossRef]
11. Cabrera-Chávez, F.; Granda-Restrepo, D.M.; Arámburo-Gálvez, J.G.; Franco-Aguilar, A.; Magaña-Ordorica, D.; de Jesús Vergara-Jiménez, M.; Ontiveros, N. Self-reported prevalence of gluten-related disorders and adherence to gluten-free diet in colombian adult population. *Gastroenterol. Res. Pract.* **2016**, *2016*, 4704309. [CrossRef] [PubMed]

12. Ontiveros, N.; Rodríguez-Bellegarrigue, C.I.; Galicia-Rodríguez, G.; de Jesús Vergara-Jiménez, M.; Zepeda-Gómez, E.M.; Arámburo-Galvez, J.G.; Gracia-Valenzuela, M.H.; Cabrera-Chávez, F. Prevalence of self-reported gluten-related disorders and adherence to a gluten-free diet in salvadoran adult population. *Int. J. Environ. Res. Public Health* **2018**, *15*, 786. [CrossRef] [PubMed]
13. Cabrera-Chávez, F.; Dezar, G.V.A.; Islas-Zamorano, A.P.; Espinoza-Alderete, J.G.; Vergara-Jiménez, M.J.; Magaña-Ordorica, D.; Ontiveros, N. Prevalence of self-reported gluten sensitivity and adherence to a gluten-free diet in argentinian adult population. *Nutrients* **2017**, *9*, 81. [CrossRef] [PubMed]
14. Volta, U.; Bardella, M.T.; Calabrò, A.; Troncone, R.; Corazza, G.R. An Italian prospective multicenter survey on patients suspected of having non-celiac gluten sensitivity. *BMC Med.* **2014**, *12*, 85. [CrossRef] [PubMed]
15. Gadelha De Mattos, Y.A.; Zandonadi, R.P.; Gandolfi, L.; Pratesi, R.; Nakano, E.Y.; Pratesi, C.B. Self-reported non-celiac gluten sensitivity in Brazil: Translation, cultural adaptation, and validation of Italian questionnaire. *Nutrients* **2019**, *11*, 781. [CrossRef]
16. Gusi, N.; Badía, X.; Herdman, M.; Olivares, P.R. Traducción y adaptación cultural de la versión española del cuestionario EQ-5D-Y en niños y adolescentes. *Aten. Primaria* **2009**, *41*, 19–23. [CrossRef] [PubMed]
17. Casellas, F.; Rodrigo, L.; Molina-Infante, J.; Vivas, S.; Lucendo, A.J.; Rosinach, M.; Dueñas, C.; Fernández-Bañares, F.; López-Vivancos, J. Transcultural adaptation and validation of the Celiac Disease Quality of Life (CD-QOL) survey, a specific questionnaire to measure quality of life in patients with celiac disease. *Rev. Española Enferm. Dig.* **2013**, *105*, 585–593. [CrossRef]
18. Henriques, E.R. Text intercomprehension by native speakers of portuguese and spanish. *DELTA* **2000**, *16*, 263–295. [CrossRef]
19. Paegelow, R.S. Back translation revisited: Differences that matter (and those that do not). *ATA Chron.* **2008**, *1*, 22.
20. Chen, H.Y.; Boore, J.R.P. Translation and back-translation in qualitative nursing research: Methodological review. *J. Clin. Nurs.* **2010**, *19*, 234–239. [CrossRef]
21. Kazi, A.M.; Khalid, W. Questionnaire designing and validation. *J. Pak. Med. Assoc.* **2012**, *62*, 514–516. [PubMed]
22. Schmidt, R.C. Managing Delphi surveys using nonparametric statistical techniques. *Decis. Sci.* **1997**, *28*, 763–774. [CrossRef]
23. Landis, J.R.; Koch, G.G. An application of hierarchical kappa-type statistics in the assessment of majority agreement among multiple observers. *Biometrics* **1977**, *33*, 363–374. [CrossRef] [PubMed]
24. Van Mol, C. Improving web survey efficiency: The impact of an extra reminder and reminder content on web survey response. *Int. J. Soc. Res. Methodol.* **2016**, *20*, 317–327. [CrossRef]

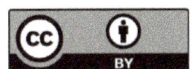

© 2019 by the authors. Licensee MDPI, Basel, Switzerland. This article is an open access article distributed under the terms and conditions of the Creative Commons Attribution (CC BY) license (http://creativecommons.org/licenses/by/4.0/).

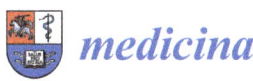

Article

Celiac-Related Autoantibodies and IL-17A in Bulgarian Patients with Dermatitis Herpetiformis: A Cross-Sectional Study

Tsvetelina Velikova [1], Martin Shahid [2], Ekaterina Ivanova-Todorova [3], Kossara Drenovska [2], Kalina Tumangelova-Yuzeir [3], Iskra Altankova [1] and Snejina Vassileva [2,*]

1. Clinical Immunology, University Hospital Lozenetz, 1407 Sofia, Bulgaria; tsvelikova@medfac.mu-sofia.bg (T.V.); altankova@abv.bg (I.A.)
2. Department of Dermatology, Faculty of Medicine, Medical University—Sofia, 1431 Sofia, Bulgaria; martin.shahidmd@gmail.com (M.S.); kosara@lycos.com (K.D.)
3. Laboratory of Clinical Immunology—University Hospital St. Ivan Rilski, 1431 Sofia, Bulgaria; katty_iv@yahoo.com (E.I.-T.); kullhem000@gmail.com (K.T.-Y.)
* Correspondence: snejina.vassileva@gmail.com; Tel.: +359-88-8565564

Received: 4 February 2019; Accepted: 10 May 2019; Published: 15 May 2019

Abstract: *Background and objectives*: Dermatitis herpetiformis (DH) is a blistering dermatosis, which shares common immunologic features with celiac disease (CD). The aim of the present study was to explore the performance of a panel of CD-related antibodies and IL-17A in Bulgarian patients with DH. *Materials and Methods:* Serum samples from 26 DH patients at mean age 53 ± 15 years and 20 healthy controls were assessed for anti-tissue transglutaminase (anti-tTG), anti-deamidated gliadin peptides (anti-DGP), anti-actin antibodies (AAA), and IL 17A by enzyme linked immuno-sorbent assay (ELISA), as well as anti-tTG, anti-gliadin (AGA), and anti-Saccharomyces cerevisiae antibodies (ASCA) using immunoblot. *Results:* The average serum levels of anti-tTG, anti-DGP, AGA, AAA, and the cytokine IL-17A were at significantly higher levels in patients with DH compared to the average levels in healthy persons which stayed below the cut-off value ($p < 0.05$). Anti-DGP and anti-tTG antibodies showed the highest diagnostic sensitivity and specificity, as well as acceptable positive and negative predictive value. None of the healthy individuals was found positive for the tested antibodies, as well as for ASCA within the DH group. All tests showed good to excellent correlations ($r = 0.5 \div 0.9$, $p < 0.01$). *Conclusions:* Although the diagnosis of DH relies on skin biopsy for histology and DIF, serologic testing of a panel of celiac-related antibodies could be employed with advantages in the diagnosing process of DH patients. Furthermore, DH patients who are positive for the investigated serologic parameters could have routine monitoring for gastrointestinal complications typical for the gluten-sensitive enteropathy.

Keywords: dermatitis herpetiformis; anti-tTG; anti-DGP; AAA; AGA; IL-17A

---

1. Introduction

Dermatitis herpetiformis (DH), also known as Duhring-Brocq disease, is a rare subepidermal blistering dermatosis, currently regarded as the specific extraintestinal manifestation of celiac disease (CD) [1,2]. It most commonly affects the skin, while associated gluten sensitive enteropathy (GSE) can be clinically variable to absent. Histologically, DH is characterized by subepidermal blisters with predominant neutrophilic infiltration in the papillary dermis. A pathognomonic finding in DH, detected by direct immunofluorescence (DIF) microscopy on perilesional uninvolved skin, is the presence of granular deposits of immunoglobulin A (IgA) along the dermo-epidermal junction (DEJ) and at the tips of the dermal papillae. Recently, it has been documented that the autoantigen for deposited cutaneous IgA is epidermal transglutaminase (eTG, TG3)—an enzyme closely related, but not identical to the tissue transglutaminase (tTG, TG2) autoantigen-specific for CD [3]. IgA deposits in skin represent antibodies against gut tTG that cross-react with the highly homologous eTG by forming insoluble aggregates in the papillary dermis [4].

The pathophysiology of DH is closely related to that of CD and involves a complex interplay among genetic, environmental, and immune factors. Both diseases occur in gluten-sensitive individuals, heal with a gluten-free diet (GFD), and relapse on gluten challenge [5]. DH and CD share the same genetic background with a high frequency of human leukocyte antigen (HLA)-DQ2 and HLA-DQ8 haplotypes [6,7]. The majority of patients with DH exhibit morphologic small-bowel changes characteristics of CD, ranging from slight villous atrophy to increased density of intraepithelial lymphocytes [1,8]. However, overt enteropathy is reported in less than 10% of patients, and the gastrointestinal symptoms are usually absent or so mild that the DH patients are unaware of them [9]. Last but not least, patients with DH and CD often have the same associated autoimmune diseases, such as juvenile diabetes, hypothyroidism, pernicious anemia, and connective tissue disorders [5].

A hallmark of CD is the loss of tolerance to wheat gluten with enhanced production of various gluten-dependent autoantibodies, as a result from the gluten-induced small-bowel mucosal T-cell activation, which is the cornerstone in the pathogenesis of the celiac pathology [10]. These circulating CD-specific antibodies are widely used to diagnose GSE serologically before proceeding to small-bowel mucosal biopsies. Historically, among the first serum-based antibody tests introduced in CD diagnostics are the antigliadin antibody (AGA) [11,12], the gluten-dependent IgA-class R1-type reticulin (ARA) [13], and endomysial autoantibody (EMA) assays [14]. In 1997, Dieterich and co-workers identified TG2 as the autoantigen of CD [15]. As various TG2-based enzyme-linked immunosorbent assays (ELISA) became available, a new era in celiac disease case finding by serology began [16]. Later research has shown that TG2 was also the specific protein antigen in the ARA and EMA tests [17]. As a result of the constant development of serologic tests for CD, a new generation of assays detecting the presence of antibodies against deamidated gliadin peptides (DGPs) as antigens appeared [18,19]. The accurate diagnosis of DH is essential, similar to CD, as the disease requires a lifelong commitment to a GFD. It relies on few but essential specific criteria, including clinical, histologic, immunopathologic, and serologic celiac-related markers, the latter being detected in DH patients as well [2,20]. Perilesional biopsy with a specific DIF microscopy finding has remained the gold standard along with the presence of suggestive clinical picture and supportive serological results [21].

Furthermore, the predictive accuracy of serological tests depends on the disease prevalence in the population [22]. In this regard, it is of interest to analyze the performance of celiac-related tests in patients from different countries and origin. In a previous report of a series of 78 DH patients from Bulgaria, the prevalence of DH among other autoimmune blistering diseases was 7.45% with a minimum estimated incidence of 0.88 cases per million annually [23].

An early event in blister formation in DH is the accumulation of neutrophils in the papillary dermis, the upregulation of the adhesion molecules, and release of enzymes and inflammatory mediators causing basement membrane damage and subsequent clefting, which could also explain the typical distribution of skin lesions at sites of trauma [24]. Interleukin (IL)-17A is involved in the production of other pro-inflammatory cytokines and matrix metalloproteinases, as well as in the attraction of neutrophils implicated in the pathogenesis of DH [25]. However, the suggested hypothesis for the role of IL-17A in DH pathogenesis needs further investigation.

Our study aimed to explore comparatively the performance of a panel of celiac-related antibodies, such as anti-tTG, AGA, anti-DGP, anti-actin (AAA) antibodies, as well as cytokine IL-17A, in a cross-sectional study of a Bulgarian cohort of DH patients.

2. Material and Methods

2.1. Serum Samples

Sera from 26 newly diagnosed and untreated DH patients (mean age 53 ± 15 years; range 18–72 years) were collected before initiation of a gluten-free diet. All patients attended the Department of Dermatology, Aleksandrovska University Hospital, Sofia and provided written informed consent to participate in the study. The diagnosis of DH was based on (i) clinical presentation and (ii) presence of granular deposits of IgA in the papillary dermis by direct IF microscopy. Sera from 20 healthy individuals at mean age 31 ± 8 (range 21–42 years) served as controls. All sera were stored at −80 °C until assayed. Female-to-male ratio for DH patients was 1:1, and for the control group 1:1.2. Age and sex differences between the studied groups were considered as non-significant ($p > 0.05$). All patients and control subjects were found negative for other autoimmune disease markers (i.e., anti-nuclear antibodies, rheumatoid factor, and anti-neutrophil cytoplasmic antibodies).

This study was performed in accordance with the declaration of Helsinki Principles and approved by the Ethical Committee of the Medical University of Sofia, Bulgaria.

2.2. Immune Serology Testing

Sera taken from all DH patients and control subjects were analyzed by ELISA and immunoblotting (Line Blot) at the Laboratory of Clinical Immunology, University Hospital "St. Ivan Rilski," Sofia.

2.2.1. Immunoenzyme Testing

ELISA commercial kits were used to determine the following celiac-related antibodies and the pro-inflammatory cytokine IL-17A:

- anti-tTG antibodies (Anti-Tissue Transglutaminase Screen IgA + IgG, Orgentec Diagnostika GmbH, cut-off value > 10 U/mL);
- anti-DGP antibodies (Quanta Lite Celiac DGP Screen IgA + IgG, Inova Diagnostics, Inc., San Diego, USA, cut-off > 15 U/mL);
- AAA (Quanta Lite F-Actin IgA ELISA, Inova Diagnostics, Inc., San Diego, USA, cut-off > 20 U/mL);
- IL-17A (Human IL-17A ELISA kit, Diaclone, GenProbe, France, sensitivity < 2.3 pg/mL).

Analyses were performed following the manufacturers' instructions.

2.2.2. Immunoblot Testing

Anti-tTG, AGA, and ASCA were assessed in serum samples by performing line blot testing (Seraline®Zöliakie-3 IgG, Seramun Diagnostica GmbH, Germany). The assay strips were scanned with IvD-registered Seraline Scan software with hardware key (Seramun Diagnostica GmbH, Germany). The results were given as the relative value of intensity.

2.3. Statistical Analysis

Row data were evaluated statistically by the software package for statistical analysis (SPSS) v.19 (SPSS®, IBM 2009). We used descriptive, correlation, and receiver operating characteristics (ROC) curve analysis to evaluate the performance characteristics of the applied tests in diagnosing DH. Results are presented as mean ± SE (standard error) or number (%). Differences between the groups were assessed using unpaired Student's T-test preceded by an evaluation of normality (Kolmogorov–Smirnoff test). The Mann–Whitney U-test was used where appropriate. A P-value of <0.05 was considered statistically significant.

3. Results

3.1. Serum Levels of the Celiac Disease-Related Autoantibodies and the Pro-Inflammatory Cytokine IL-17A

The mean ELISA values of the measured parameters in DH patients and the control group are presented on Figure 1 and Supplementary Table S1. The mean levels of anti-tTG and anti-DGP antibodies were significantly higher in DH patients compared to healthy controls (36.9 ± 20.3 IU/mL versus 2.1 ± 0.4 IU/mL, $p = 0.02$, and 40.7 ± 10.2 IU/mL versus 1.87 ± 0.68, $p < 0.001$, respectively). Similarly, the AAA titers significantly differed between both groups, being moderately higher in DH sera than in the healthy subjects (22.6 ± 3.9 IU/mL versus 9.1 ± 0.9 IU/mL, $p = 0.05$). There was a 60-fold increase in the concentrations of IL-17A in DH patients compared to control sera (5.3 ± 2.2 pg/mL versus 0.08 ± 0.07 pg/mL, $p = 0.031$) (Figure 1A).

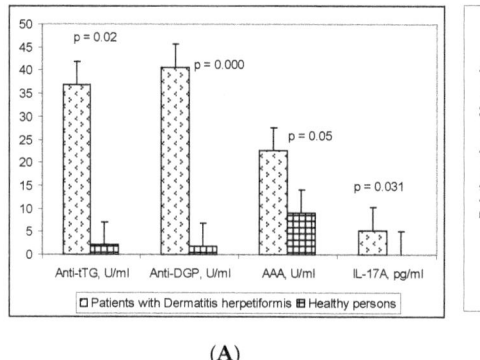
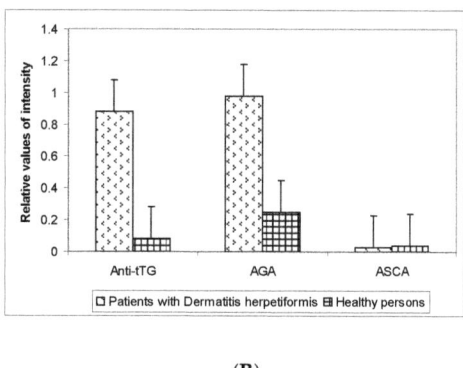

(A)   (B)

Figure 1. Mean serum levels of anti-tTG antibodies, anti-DGP, anti-actin antibodies, and IL-17A in the study groups, assessed by (**A**) ELISA and (**B**) line blot.

The mean serum levels of the autoantibodies investigated by Line blot are also demonstrated (Figure 1 and Table S1). There were significantly higher levels of anti-tTG and AGA antibodies in DH patients compared to healthy controls (0.88 ± 0.24 versus 0.08 ± 0.02, $p = 0.003$, and 0.98 ± 0.31 versus 0.25 ± 0.08, $p = 0.030$, respectively). In contrast, no differences were found in the mean levels of ASCA within the studied groups (Figure 1B).

3.2. Performance Characteristics of the Celiac-Related Antibodies Tested in DH Patients

The results of the performance of anti-tTG, anti-DGP antibodies, AAA, and AGA, assessed by ELISA and line blot are shown in Table 1. Antibodies against tTG were found in 11 (42.3%) (IgA + IgG, ELISA) and 12 (46%) (IgG, line blot) patients with DH. Half of the DH patients had AGA IgG (Line blot) in their sera, and 12 (46.4%) were positive for anti-DGP antibodies. The smallest number of patients—9 (34.7%) were found positive for AAA (ELISA).

None of the control sera were tested positive for anti-tTG (ELISA and blot), AAA or AGA, whereas one subject showed positive results for anti-DGP. This defined a specificity of 100% in distinguishing DH from healthy individuals for the test systems applied in our study, excluding anti-DGP antibodies, which exerted a specificity of 95%.

Positive predictive values (PPV) for all tests were 100%, except for anti-DGP—90.9%. The negative predictive values (NPV) of the test remained slightly above 50%, and the highest NPV was observed for AGA (60%) and anti-tTG (Line blot) (59%).

Table 1. Performance characteristics of anti-tTG antibodies, anti-DGP antibodies, AAA, and AGA, assessed by ELISA and line blot in Dermatitis Herpetiformis patients.

	Anti-tTG IgA + IgG (ELISA)	Anti-DGP IgA + IgG (ELISA)	AAA IgG (ELISA)	Anti-tTG IgG (Line Blot)	AGA IgG (Line Blot)
Sensitivity	42.3%	46.4%	34.7%	46%	50%
Specificity	100%	95%	100%	100%	100%
PPV *	100%	90.9%	100%	100%	100%
NPV **	57%	57.1%	54.1%	59%	60%

* PPV, positive predictive value; ** NPV, negative predictive value.

3.3. ROC Curve Analysis of the Celiac Disease-Related Antibodies and IL-17A in DH Patients

The ROC curve analyses of the ELISA tests revealed the best performance of anti-DGP antibodies (AUC 0.939, $p < 0.001$), followed by anti-tTG antibodies testing (AUC 0.864, $p = 0.002$) (Supplementary Table S2). We did not find significant AUC for AAA. According to IL-17 serum levels, our results demonstrated excellent performance of the test (AUC 0.811, $p < 0.05$) (Figure 2A). From the celiac-related antibodies assessed by line blot, anti-tTG testing alone had significant AUC of 0.734, while the other tests showed unsatisfactory performance (Figure 2B).

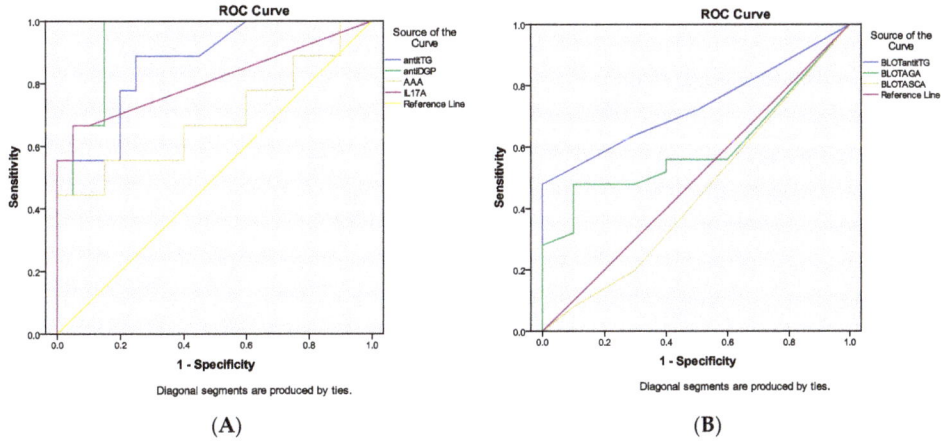

Figure 2. Receiver operating characteristics (ROC) curve analysis of the tested parameters, assessed by (**A**) ELISA and (**B**) line blot.

3.4. Correlation between Tests

The results of all tests showed good to excellent correlation to each other ($r = 0.5 \div 0.9$, $p < 0.01$) (Table 2). The strongest correlations were established for the following pairs of antibodies, all of them assessed by ELISA: anti-tTG—IL-17A ($r = 0.938$, $p < 0.001$), anti-tTG – anti-DGP ($r = 0.894$, $p < 0.001$), and anti-tTG—AAA ($r = 0.863$, $p = 0.001$). In comparison, the correlation between anti-DGP antibodies and IL-17A was evaluated as a weak one ($r = 0.452$, $p = 0.031$). Anti-tTG ELISA levels moderately correlated with anti-tTG assessed by line blot ($r = 0.520$, $p = 0.003$) (Table 2).

Table 2. Correlation between tests. Results are presented as Pearson's coefficient (r) and significance (p).

	Anti-tTG (ELISA)	Anti-DGP (ELISA)	AAA (ELISA)	IL-17A (ELISA)	Anti-tTG (Line Blot)	AGA (Line Blot)
Anti-tTG (ELISA)		r = 0.894 $p < 0.001$	r = 0.863 $p = 0.001$	r = 0.938 $p < 0.001$	r = 0.520 $p = 0.003$	r = 0.507 $p = 0.076$
	anti-DGP (ELISA)		r = 0.502 $p = 0.009$	r = 0.452 $p = 0.031$	r = 0.532 $p = 0.001$	r = 0.346 $p = 0.038$
		AAA (ELISA)		r = 0.692 $p < 0.001$	r = 0.112 $p = 0.500$	r = 0.221 $p = 0.186$
			IL-17A(ELISA)		r = 0.079 $p = 0.676$	r = −0.222 $p = 0.238$
				Anti-tTG (Line blot)		r = 0.678 $p < 0.001$
					AGA (Line blot)	

All Pearson's coefficients were calculated by bivariate correlation, except for the line blot results where the Spearman coefficient was calculated via Chi-square test.

4. Discussion

Growing evidence shows that patients with DH may possess most of the specific autoantibodies that can be found in patients with CD, including circulating autoantibodies against gliadin, tTG, and DGP [1]. On the other hand, conflicting results were obtained by the use of the anti-DGP ELISA for detecting gluten enteropathy in DH patients. Previously reported sensitivities for IgA anti-DGP antibodies vary from 46% to 78% [20,26]. In this study, the relative sensitivities and specificities of a panel of CD-related autoantibodies in Bulgarian patients with DH were compared with the reactivities of control healthy subjects. We included conventional celiac-related antibodies—anti-tTG, anti-DGP, and AGA, as well as AAA, the latter being used for non-invasive evaluation of villous atrophy. ASCA were tested along with other antibodies due to the presence of coated Mannan on the Line blot. Moreover, we were interested in assessing the serum levels of IL-17A in DH patients. We chose not to compare EMA with the other autoantibodies in our celiac-related panel due to the subjective semiquantitative nature of EMA testing that is not easy to standardize.

All investigated celiac-related antibodies—anti-tTG, anti-DGP, and AGA, independent of the used method (ELISA or Line blot), were significantly higher in the DH group compared to the healthy controls. Nevertheless, the sensitivity and specificity of the applied tests were acceptable. We found that 42.3% of our DH patients were positive for anti-tTG (IgA + IgG) assessed by ELISA. When we tested the serum samples for IgG anti-tTG by line blot, we found a higher sensitivity of 46%. Half of the DH patients had IgG AGA (Line blot) in their serum samples, and 46.4% had anti-DGP (ELISA) antibodies. We also defined the specificity of 100% for anti-tTG (ELISA and line blot), AAA, and AGA in discriminating DH from healthy persons, as well as a specificity of 95% for anti-DGP antibodies. These results are in accordance with other studies, demonstrating sensitivity ranges between 47% and 100% and specificity ranging 90% to 100% for celiac-related antibodies in patients with DH [9,27–32]. PPVs for all tests were 100%, except for anti-DGP, which was 90.9% due to one positive healthy individual. Unfortunately, the NPVs of the tests remained slightly above 50%, and the highest NPV was observed for AGA (60%) and anti-tTG (59%) assessed by line blot. However, during the last decade, only a few studies updated this information. Thus, our results contribute to previously published literature data.

Comparing tests by the ROC curve analyses, the best performance was revealed for anti-DGP antibodies, followed by anti-tTG (ELISA) testing and anti-tTG (Line blot) antibodies. Although the specificity of AGA was 50%, the AUC of 0.600 was non-significant and therefore, unreliable.

Among all celiac-related serological tests, IgA anti-tTG antibodies have been considered the most sensitive and specific ones that should be tested in patients with DH symptoms [1]. Since some patients with DH or CD may have selective IgA deficiency, we chose the dual IgG/IgA test system to exclude false-negative results. [27,33]. In our study, the performance of anti-DGP in diagnosing DH was shown to be superior to the anti-tTG antibodies. In previous comparative studies among DH patients, the sensitivity and specificity of anti-DGP were either lower than those of anti-tTG and EMA, similar, or superior to them [34], as it is in the present study. The possible explanations for such discrepancies lie in the fact that anti-DGP and AGA, which are directed against deamidated gliadin peptides and whole gliadin peptide, respectively, are related to the presence of intestinal damage, whereas antibodies against the converting enzyme tTG are linked not only to mucosal but also to skin lesions as well [34]. However, current knowledge has shown that the available serologic armamentarium lacks sensitivity when used in patients with mild or minor enteropathy [35,36]. The similarity of DH and CD related to the enteropathy makes DH a fascinating model of skin CD, where papulovesicular and pruritic rash can be concomitant with a broad spectrum of intestinal damage varying from normal structure to villous atrophy [37]. However, DH is the second gluten-sensitive disorder exhibiting varied histological damage where one can assess the performance of the celiac serology [34]. In the present study, we chose to assess by ELISA anti-tTG and anti-DGP antibodies of both IgA and IgG subclasses. The results obtained allowed us to conclude that the combination of both isotypes of anti-DGP assays has higher specificity than IgA anti-tTG.

There is an insufficient number of investigations regarding anti-actin testing in DH patients. Of the 26 patients with DH in our study, nine were positive for AAA. However, no significant differences were found in the serum levels of AAA in DH patients and healthy controls. Serum levels of IgG AAA were assessed by ELISA in a single study on a series of 10 adult Romanian DH patients. The authors documented sensitivity and specificity of 33.3% and 100%, respectively, for AAA in DH patients [38]. Our results also showed that the AUC for AAA was unacceptable and therefore not reliable for the DH diagnosis.

We did not find differences in the mean levels of ASCA within the studied groups. Although ASCA have been reported to be positive in about 30% of CD patients [39], which was also confirmed by us in a cohort of Bulgarian CD patients [40], there were no data regarding ASCA in DH patients available so far.

Concerning the IL-17A, in a single study Zebrowska et al. documented significantly higher expression of this cytokine in the epidermis (perilesional skin) and the serum of DH and bullous pemphigoid patients, compared to the control group [41]. We also detected 60-fold higher concentrations of IL-17A in DH patients compared to healthy controls ($p = 0.031$). Two studies provided data for the involvement of IL-17A in DH pathogenesis. Juczynska et al. demonstrated increased expression of JAK/STAT proteins in skin lesions in patients with DH and bullous pemphigoid in comparison to perilesional skin and control group [42]. They suggested that pro-inflammatory cytokine network and induction of inflammatory infiltrate in tissues can contribute to the pathogenesis of skin lesions in both diseases. Surprisingly, serum IL-17 demonstrated excellent performance in our study (AUC 0.811, $p = 0.008$), which could be of benefit for the clinical practice.

We found good to excellent correlation ($r = 0.5 \div 0.9$, $p < 0.01$) between the tests. The strongest correlations were established for the following pairs: anti-tTG (ELISA)—IL-17A, anti-tTG (ELISA)—anti-DGP antibodies, and anti-tTG (ELISA)—AAA. These results suggested a good coincidence between the different tests in diagnosing DH. There was a moderate correlation between anti-tTG antibodies estimated by ELISA and by line blot, which is not encouraging regarding the interchangeability between the two methods for anti-tTG detection. Previous studies showed similar correlations between celiac-related antibodies in patients with GSE [40].

This study has some limitations. The relatively small size of the study population might have affected the significance of the results. The lack of data on anti-TG3 is another weak point of the present work. We assume that further research involving a larger number of DH patients and newly emerging test systems for detection of other transglutaminase antibodies (TG3 and/or TG6) would clarify the findings presented in the current study and may have a significant impact on the clinical practice.

5. Conclusions

Serologic tests are important noninvasive screening tool among symptomatic patients with clinical suspicion of DH that can help select patients for diagnostic DIF analysis. Furthermore, such tests are helpful in the resolution of ambiguous and false-negative DIF results. The usability of serologic DH tests is defined by their sensitivity and specificity, which are quite variable based on current data. This is due to scarcity of data from limited populations.

In this respect, serologic testing with a panel of celiac-related antibodies, rather than individual ones, may be successfully employed to support the diagnosis of DH. In our study, the performance of anti-DGP in diagnosing DH was shown to be superior to that of anti-tTG antibodies. In addition, the best performance (ROC curve analysis) was revealed for anti-DGP antibodies followed by anti-tTG ELISA. This is the first such study among Bulgarian patients and hopefully more will follow. Further studies among different populations are needed in order to improve evidence-based results and to decrease interpolation of data.

Supplementary Materials: The following are available online at http://www.mdpi.com/1010-660X/55/5/136/s1, Table S1: Serum levels of the celiac-related antibodies and IL-17A in DH patients and controls, investigated by ELISA and immunoblot. Results are presented as Mean ± SE (Range). Table S2: Receiver operating characteristics (ROC) curve analysis of the tested parameters assessed by ELISA and line blot.

Author Contributions: Conceptualization: T.V., I.A., and S.V.; data curation: T.V. and K.D.; Formal analysis: T.V., M.S., K.T.-Y., I.A. and S.V.; funding acquisition, T.V. and I.A.; investigation: T.V., K.T.-Y. and I.A.; methodology, T.V., E.I.-T., K.T.-Y., I.A. and S.V.; project administration: T.V. and I.A.; resources: M.S., K.D. and S.V.; supervision: T.V., I.A. and S.V.; validation: T.V. and I.A.; visualization: T.V.; writing—original draft: T.V.; writing—review and editing: M.S., E.I.-T., K.D., I.A. and S.V.

Acknowledgments: This study was supported by grant number 12-D/2013-2014, project № 3-D, from the Medical University, Sofia.

Conflicts of Interest: The authors declare no conflict of interest. The founding sponsors had no role in the design of the study; in the collection, analyses, or interpretation of data; in the writing of the manuscript, and in the decision to publish the results.

References

1. Antiga, E.; Caproni, M. The diagnosis and treatment of dermatitis herpetiformis. *Clin. Cosmet. Investig. Dermatol.* **2015**, *8*, 257–265. [CrossRef] [PubMed]
2. Caproni, M.; Antiga, E.; Melani, L.; Fabbri, P. The Italian Group for Cutaneous Immunopathology. Guidelines for the diagnosis and treatment of dermatitis herpetiformis. *J. Eur. Acad. Dermatol. Venereol.* **2009**, *23*, 633–638. [CrossRef] [PubMed]
3. Reunala, T.; Salmi, T.T.; Hervonen, K.; Kaukinen, K.; Collin, P. Dermatitis Herpetiformis: A Common Extraintestinal Manifestation of Coeliac Disease. *Nutrients* **2018**, *10*, 602. [CrossRef] [PubMed]
4. Sárdy, M.; Kárpáti, S.; Merkl, B.; Paulsson, M.; Smyth, N. Epidermal transglutaminase (TGase 3) is the autoantigen of dermatitis herpetiformis. *J. Exp. Med.* **2002**, *195*, 747–757. [CrossRef] [PubMed]
5. Collin, P.; Salmi, T.T.; Hervonen, K.; Kaukinen, K.; Reunala, T. Dermatitis herpetiformis: A cutaneous manifestation of coeliac disease. *Ann. Med.* **2017**, *49*, 23–31. [CrossRef] [PubMed]
6. Bonciani, D.; Verdelli, A.; Bonciolini, V.; D'Errico, A.; Antiga, E.; Fabbri, P.; Caproni, M. Dermatitis herpetiformis: From the genetics to the development of skin lesions. *Clin. Dev. Immunol.* **2012**, *2012*, 239691. [CrossRef]
7. Reunala, T. Dermatitis herpetiformis: Coeliac disease of the skin. *Ann. Med.* **1998**, *30*, 416–418. [CrossRef]
8. Savilahti, E.; Reunala, T.; Mäki, M. Increase of lymphocytes bearing the gamma/delta T cell receptor in the jejunum of patients with dermatitis herpetiformis. *Gut* **1992**, *33*, 206–211. [CrossRef]

9. Alonso-Llamazares, J.; Gibson, L.E.; Rogers, R.S. Clinical, pathologic, and immunopathologic features of dermatitis herpetiformis: Review of the Mayo Clinic experience. *Int. J. Dermatol.* **2007**, *46*, 910–919. [CrossRef]
10. Mazzarella, G. Effector and suppressor T cells in celiac disease. *World J. Gastroenterol.* **2015**, *21*, 7349–7356. [CrossRef]
11. Berger, E. *Zur Allergischen Pathogenese der Cöliakie*; Bibliotheca Paediatrica; S Karger Ag: Basel, Switzerland, 1958; pp. 1–55.
12. Rossi, T.M.; Tjota, A. Serologic indicators of celiac disease. *J. Pediatr. Gastroenterol. Nutr.* **1998**, *26*, 205–210. [CrossRef] [PubMed]
13. Seah, P.P.; Fry, L.; Hoffbrand, A.V.; Holborow, E.J. Tissue antibodies in dermatitis herpetiformis and adult coeliac disease. *Lancet* **1971**, *1*, 834–836. [CrossRef]
14. Chorzelski, T.P.; Beutner, E.H.; Sulej, J.; Tchorzewska, H.; Jablonska, S.; Kumar, V.; Kapuscinska, A. IgA anti-endomysium antibody. A new immunological marker of dermatitis herpetiformis and coeliac disease. *Br. J. Dermatol.* **1984**, *111*, 395–402. [CrossRef] [PubMed]
15. Dieterich, W.; Ehnis, T.; Bauer, M.; Donner, P.; Volta, U.; Riecken, E.O.; Schuppan, D. Identification of tissue transglutaminase as the autoantigen of celiac disease. *Nat. Med.* **1997**, *3*, 797–801. [CrossRef] [PubMed]
16. Caja, S.; Mäki, M.; Kaukinen, K.; Lindfors, K. Antibodies in celiac disease: Implications beyond diagnostics. *Cell. Mol. Immunol.* **2011**, *8*, 103–109. [CrossRef]
17. Korponay-Szabó, I.R.; Laurila, K.; Szondy, Z.; Halttunen, T.; Szalai, Z.; Dahlbom, I.; Rantala, I.; Kovács, J.B.; Fésüs, L.; Mäki, M. Missing endomysial and reticulin binding of coeliac antibodies in transglutaminase 2 knockout tissues. *Gut* **2003**, *52*, 199–204. [CrossRef] [PubMed]
18. Molberg, O.; Mcadam, S.N.; Körner, R.; Quarsten, H.; Kristiansen, C.; Madsen, L.; Fugger, L.; Scott, H.; Norén, O.; Roepstorff, P.; et al. Tissue transglutaminase selectively modifies gliadin peptides that are recognized by gut-derived T cells in celiac disease. *Nat. Med.* **1998**, *4*, 713–717. [CrossRef]
19. Kasperkiewicz, M.; Dähnrich, C.; Probst, C.; Komorowski, L.; Stöcker, W.; Schlumberger, W.; Zillikens, D.; Rose, C. Novel assay for detecting celiac disease-associated autoantibodies in dermatitis herpetiformis using deamidated gliadin-analogous fusion peptides. *J. Am. Acad. Dermatol.* **2012**, *66*, 583–588. [CrossRef] [PubMed]
20. Sugai, E.; Smecuol, E.; Niveloni, S.; Vázquez, H.; Label, M.; Mazure, R.; Czech, A.; Kogan, Z.; Mauriño, E.; Bai, J.C. Celiac disease serology in dermatitis herpetiformis. Which is the best option for detecting gluten sensitivity? *Acta Gastroenterol. Latinoam.* **2006**, *36*, 197–201.
21. Fuertes, I.; Mascaró, J.M.; Bombí, J.A.; Iranzo, P. A Retrospective Study of Clinical, Histological, and Immunological Characteristics in Patients with Dermatitis Herpetiformis. The Experience of Hospital Clinic de Barcelona, Spain between 1995 and 2010 and a Review of the Literature. *Actas Dermo-Sifiliográficas Engl. Ed.* **2011**, *102*, 699–705. [CrossRef]
22. Dahele, A.; Gosh, S. The role of serological tests in redefining coeliac disease. *Proc. R. Coll. Phys. Edinb.* **2000**, *30*, 100–113.
23. Shahid, M.; Drenovska, K.; Velikova, T.; Vassileva, S. Dermatitis herpetiformis in Bulgaria: Report of 78 patients. *J. Investig. Dermatol.* **2017**, *137*, S280. [CrossRef]
24. Clarindo, M.V.; Possebon, A.T.; Soligo, E.M.; Uyeda, H.; Ruaro, R.T.; Empinotti, J.C. Dermatitis herpetiformis: Pathophysiology, clinical presentation, diagnosis and treatment. *An. Bras. Dermatol.* **2014**, *89*, 865–877. [CrossRef]
25. Harrington, L.E.; Hatton, R.D.; Mangan, P.R.; Turner, H.; Murphy, T.L.; Murphy, K.M.; Weaver, C.T. Interleukin 17-producing CD4+ effector T cells develop via a lineage distinct from the T helper type 1 and 2 lineages. *Nat. Immunol.* **2005**, *6*, 1123–1132. [CrossRef]
26. Jaskowski, T.D.; Donaldson, M.R.; Hull, C.M.; Wilson, A.R.; Hill, H.R.; Zone, J.J.; Book, L.S. Novel Screening Assay Performance in Pediatric Celiac Disease and Adult Dermatitis Herpetiformis. *J. Pediatr. Gastroenterol. Nutr.* **2010**, *51*, 19–23. [CrossRef]
27. Desai, A.M.; Krishnan, R.S.; Hsu, S. Medical pearl: Using tissue transglutaminase antibodies to diagnose dermatitis herpetiformis. *J. Am. Acad. Dermatol.* **2005**, *53*, 867–868. [CrossRef]
28. Porter, W.M.; Unsworth, D.J.; Lock, R.J.; Hardman, C.M.; Baker, B.S.; Fry, L. Tissue transglutaminase antibodies in dermatitis herpetiformis. *Gastroenterology* **1999**, *117*, 749–750. [CrossRef]

29. Dieterich, W.; Schuppan, D.; Laag, E.; Bruckner-Tuderman, L.; Reunala, T.; Kárpáti, S.; Zágoni, T.; Riecken, E.O. Antibodies to Tissue Transglutaminase as Serologic Markers in Patients with Dermatitis Herpetiformis. *J. Investig. Dermatol.* **1999**, *113*, 133–136. [CrossRef]
30. Kumar, V.; Jarzabek-Chorzelska, M.; Sulej, J.; Rajadhyaksha, M.; Jablonska, S. Tissue Transglutaminase and Endomysial Antibodies—Diagnostic Markers of Gluten-Sensitive Enteropathy in Dermatitis Herpetiformis. *Clin. Immunol.* **2001**, *98*, 378–382. [CrossRef]
31. Koop, I.; Ilchmann, R.; Izzi, L.; Adragna, A.; Koop, H.; Barthelmes, H. Detection of autoantibodies against tissue transglutaminase in patients with celiac disease and dermatitis herpetiformis. *Am. J. Gastroenterol.* **2000**, *95*, 2009–2014. [CrossRef]
32. Caproni, M.; Cardinali, C.; Renzi, D.; Calabrò, A.; Fabbri, P. Tissue transglutaminase antibody assessment in dermatitis herpetiformis. *Br. J. Dermatol.* **2001**, *144*, 196–197. [CrossRef]
33. Sárdy, M.; Csikós, M.; Geisen, C.; Preisz, K.; Kornseé, Z.; Tomsits, E.; Töx, U.; Hunzelmann, N.; Wieslander, J.; Kárpáti, S.; et al. Tissue transglutaminase ELISA positivity in autoimmune disease independent of gluten-sensitive disease. *Clin. Chim. Acta Int. J. Clin. Chem.* **2007**, *376*, 126–135. [CrossRef]
34. Sugai, E.; Hwang, H.J.; Vazquez, H.; Smecuol, E.; Niveloni, S.; Mazure, R.; Maurino, E.; Aeschlimann, P.; Binder, W.; Aeschlimann, D.; et al. New Serology Assays Can Detect Gluten Sensitivity among Enteropathy Patients Seronegative for Anti-Tissue Transglutaminase. *Clin. Chem.* **2010**, *56*, 661–665. [CrossRef] [PubMed]
35. Green, P.H.R.; Rostami, K.; Marsh, M.N. Diagnosis of coeliac disease. *Best Pract. Res. Clin. Gastroenterol.* **2005**, *19*, 389–400. [CrossRef]
36. Rostami, K.; Kerckhaert, J.; Tiemessen, R.; von Blomberg, B.M.; Meijer, J.W.; Mulder, C.J. Sensitivity of antiendomysium and antigliadin antibodies in untreated celiac disease: Disappointing in clinical practice. *Am. J. Gastroenterol.* **1999**, *94*, 888–894. [CrossRef]
37. Marsh, M.N. Gluten, major histocompatibility complex, and the small intestine. A molecular and immunobiologic approach to the spectrum of gluten sensitivity ('celiac sprue'). *Gastroenterology* **1992**, *102*, 330–354. [CrossRef]
38. Samaşca, G.; Băican, A.; Pop, T.; Pîrvan, A.; Miu, N.; Andreica, M.; Cristea, V.; Dejica, D. IgG-F-actin antibodies in celiac disease and dermatitis herpetiformis. *Rom. Arch.* **2010**, *69*, 177–182.
39. Granito, A.; Muratori, L.; Muratori, P.; Guidi, M.; Lenzi, M.; Bianchi, F.B.; Volta, U. Anti-saccharomyces cerevisiae antibodies (ASCA) in coeliac disease. *Gut* **2006**, *55*, 296.
40. Velikova, T.; Spassova, Z.; Tumangelova-Yuzeir, K.; Krasimirova, E.; Ivanova-Todorova, E.; Kyurkchiev, D.; Altankova, I. Serological Update on Celiac Disease Diagnostics in Adults. *Int. J. Celiac Dis.* **2018**, *6*, 20–25. [CrossRef]
41. Zebrowska, A.; Wagrowska-Danilewicz, M.; Danilewicz, M.; Stasikowska-Kanicka, O.; Cynkier, A.; Sysa-Jedrzejowska, A.; Waszczykowska, E. IL-17 Expression in Dermatitis Herpetiformis and Bullous Pemphigoid. *Mediat. Inflamm.* **2013**, *2013*, 967987. [CrossRef]
42. Juczynska, K.; Wozniacka, A.; Waszczykowska, E.; Danilewicz, M.; Wagrowska-Danilewicz, M.; Wieczfinska, J.; Pawliczak, R.; Zebrowska, A. Expression of the JAK/STAT Signaling Pathway in Bullous Pemphigoid and Dermatitis Herpetiformis. *Mediat. Inflamm.* **2017**, *2017*, 6716419. [CrossRef] [PubMed]

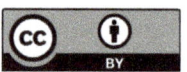

© 2019 by the authors. Licensee MDPI, Basel, Switzerland. This article is an open access article distributed under the terms and conditions of the Creative Commons Attribution (CC BY) license (http://creativecommons.org/licenses/by/4.0/).

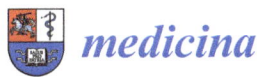

Review

The Skin in Celiac Disease Patients: The Other Side of the Coin

Ludovico Abenavoli [1,*], Stefano Dastoli [2], Luigi Bennardo [2], Luigi Boccuto [3,4], Maria Passante [2], Martina Silvestri [2], Ilaria Proietti [5], Concetta Potenza [5], Francesco Luzza [1] and Steven Paul Nisticò [2]

1. Digestive Physiopathology Unit, Department of Health Sciences, Magna Graecia University of Catanzaro, 88100 Catanzaro, Italy
2. Dermatology Unit, Department of Health Sciences, Magna Graecia University of Catanzaro, 88100 Catanzaro, Italy
3. JC Self Research Institute, Greenwood Genetic Center, Greenwood, SC 29646, USA
4. Clemson University School of Health Research, Clemson University, Clemson, SC 29634, USA
5. Dermatology Unit "Daniele Innocenzi", Department of Medical-Surgical Sciences and Biotechnologies, Sapienza University of Rome, Polo Pontino, 04110 Terracina, Italy
* Correspondence: l.abenavoli@unicz.it; Tel.: +39 0961-3694387

Received: 31 May 2019; Accepted: 5 September 2019; Published: 9 September 2019

Abstract: Celiac disease (CD) is an autoimmune enteropathy that primarily affects the small intestine and is characterized by atrophy of intestinal villi. The manifestations of the disease improve following a gluten-free diet (GFD). CD is associated with various extra-intestinal diseases. Several skin manifestations are described in CD patients. The present paper reviews all CD-associated skin diseases reported in the literature and tries to analyze the pathogenic mechanisms possibly involved in these associations. Different hypotheses have been proposed to explain the possible mechanisms involved in every association between CD and cutaneous manifestations. An abnormal small intestinal permeability seems to be implicated in various dermatological manifestations. However, most of the associations between CD and cutaneous diseases is based on case reports and case series and a few controlled studies. To better assess the real involvement of the cutaneous district in CD patients, large multicentric controlled clinical trials are required.

Keywords: gluten; gut; enteropathy; gluten-free diet; level of evidences

1. Introduction

Celiac disease (CD) is an autoimmune disorder that occurs in genetically predisposed subjects who develop an immune reaction to gluten [1]. CD primarily involves the small intestine. However, the clinical presentation can be characterized by both intestinal and extra-intestinal manifestations. The incidence of CD is up to 1% in the majority of populations. Genetic factors play an important role in the pathogenesis of CD. The almost totality of the patients with CD possess class II human leukocyte antigen (HLA) -DQ2 and -DQ8, or their variants. However, up to 40% of people with European and Asian origins carries these genes, indicating that the expression of these molecules is necessary, but not sufficient, to develop the disease [2].

The intestinal immune response to gluten is present in two sites: The lamina propria and the epithelium [3]. Both the lamina propria (adaptive) and intraepithelial (innate) immune responses are necessary for the generation of the pathological celiac lesion, but how these two processes interact is not clear [1]. The presentation of CD has shifted from the historically classic malabsorption pediatric symptoms in childhood to non-specific symptoms, which may be present also in adulthood. The symptoms classically include weight loss, chronic diarrhea, and failure to thrive. Non-specific symptoms are more common and include gastrointestinal manifestations, such as bloating, abdominal pain, constipation, as well as extra-intestinal manifestations, as osteoporosis, headache, iron deficiency, and chronic fatigue [4,5].

In the last years, skin diseases are acquiring more and more importance among the extra-intestinal manifestations of CD [4]. The aim of this review is to summarize the association between cutaneous diseases and CD. For this reason, searches were undertaken in the PubMed/Medline database in March 2019 using the following terms: A combined research of "celiac disease" and "skin", "blistering diseases", "cutaneous manifestations", "pemphigus", and other skin disorders. In this way, 7923 articles were found and 100 were selected as reported in Figure 1. In addition, the studies were rated using the Oxford Centre for Evidence Based Medicine 2011 and levels of evidence assigned to each association [6]. The assigned levels of evidence were discussed among members until consensus was reached (Table 1).

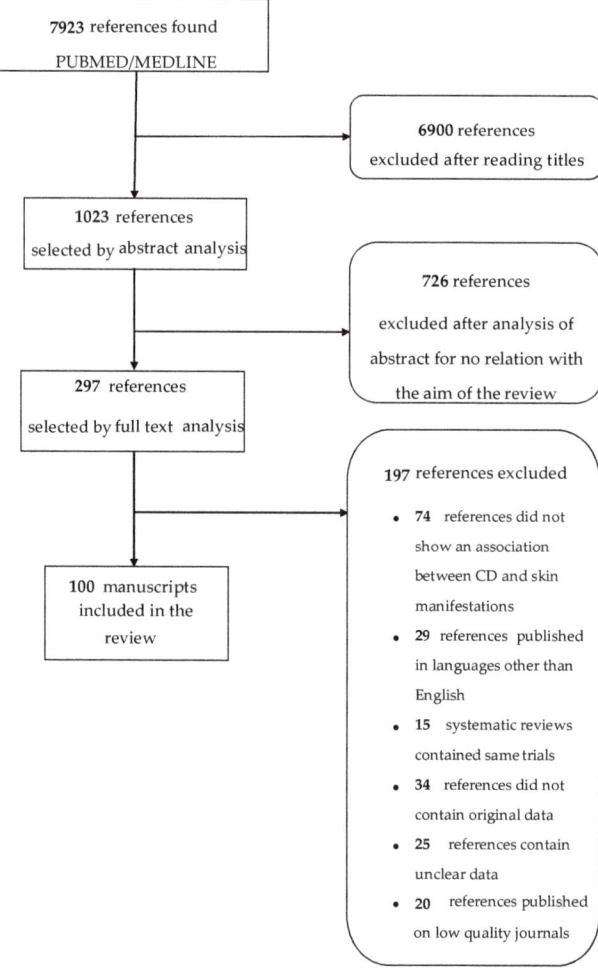

Figure 1. Flow chart of the identified and selected studies.

Table 1. Level of evidences of the association between celiac disease and skin disorders.

Disorders Associated	Level of Evidence
Pemphigus	4
Dermatitis herpetiformis	1A
Linear IgA bullous dermatosis	4
Urticaria	2B
Hereditary angioneurotic edema	4
Atopic dermatitis	4
Cutaneous vasculitis	4
Erythema nodosum	4
Erythema elevatum diutinum	4
Necrolytic migratory erythema	4
Psoriasis	1A
Vitiligo disease	3B
Stomatous Aphtitis	2A
Behçet's disease	4
Oral lichen planus	3B
Dermatomyositis	4
Porphyria	4
Rosacea	2B
Alopecia areata	3B
Acquired hypertrichosis lanuginosa	5
Pyoderma gangrenosum	4
Ichthyosiform dermatoses	4
Pellagra	5
Generalized acquired cutis laxa	5
Skin malignancies	2B

Levels of evidence: 1A Systematic Reviews of Randomized Control Trials; 1B Individual RCT; 2A Systematic Reviews of cohort studies; 2B Individual cohort study; 3A Systematic Reviews of case-control studies; 3B Individual Case-Control Study; 4 Case-series (and poor quality cohort and case-control studies); 5 Expert opinion without explicit critical appraisal.

2. Blistering Diseases

Blistering diseases are characterized by the formation of bullae, blisters, and erosions on the cutaneous surface. Among them pemphigus, dermatitis herpetiformis and linear IgA bullous dermatosis may be related to CD.

2.1. Pemphigus

Pemphigus is a group of autoimmune diseases characterized by the formation of flaccid bullae and erosions of the mucosae and skin [7]. In 2014, an association among pemphigus, epilepsy, and CD was reported [8]. Various case reports associate pemphigus with the positive blood markers of CD, and in particular IgA anti-gliadin (AGA) and anti-endomysium (EMA) antibodies [8,9]. In this case, instauration of a gluten-free diet (GFD) may induce pemphigus disappearance [9].

2.2. Dermatitis Herpetiformis

Dermatitis herpetiformis (DH) or Duhring-Brocq disease is an inflammatory skin disease characterized by a chronic relapsing course and typical histopathological and immunopathological findings. It presents as symmetrical, grouped polymorphic lesions consisting of erythema, urticarial plaques, and papules involving the extensor surfaces of the elbows, knees, shoulders, buttocks, sacral region, neck, face, and scalp. Herpetiform vesicles may occur later and are often immediately excoriated, resulting in erosions, crusted papules, or areas of post-inflammatory dyschromia. Petechial or ecchymotic lesions may occur in the palmoplantar regions and are observed more frequently in children. DH is the most common extra-intestinal manifestation of CD in >85% of cases and it improves significantly with a GFD. In fact, DH and CD share the same HLA haplotypes, DQ2 and DQ8 [10]. Various authors showed the decreasing incidence rate of DH, along with a simultaneous rapid increase in CD. This fits the hypothesis that subclinical, undiagnosed CD is a prerequisite for the development of DH [11].

Moreover, patients with DH have elevated levels of IgA anti-transglutaminase antibodies both TG2 and TG3, which are the most sensitive and specific antibodies to be tested in patients with a suspected DH [12]. At present, a valid hypothesis is that the immune pathogenesis of DH starts from hidden CD in the gut with a TG2, and possibly also a TG3, autoantibody response and evolves into an immune complex deposition of high avidity IgA TG3 antibodies together with the TG3 enzyme in the papillary dermis. This seems to be due to the active TG3 enzyme in the aggregates resulting in covalent cross-linking of the complex to the dermal structures [13].

A small bowel biopsy shows typical CD alterations in almost all these patients, including: Partial-to-total villous atrophy, elongated crypts, decreased villus/crypt ratio, increased mitotic index in the crypts, increased intraepithelial lymphocyte (IEL) density, increased IEL mitotic index, infiltration of plasma cells, lymphocytes, mast cells, and eosinophils and basophils into the lamina propria [14]. The histology of DH is characterized by subepidermal vesicles and blisters associated with the accumulation of neutrophils at the top of dermal papillae. Sometimes, eosinophils can be found within the inflammatory infiltrate, making difficult the differential diagnosis with bullous pemphigoid. The histopathology of DH is not diagnostic as other bullous diseases, including linear IgA dermatosis and epidermolysis bullosa acquisita, which may show similar histologic findings [10]. It is important to obtain a skin fragment near the vesicle for histopathological analysis to identify neutrophilic micro-abscesses. Neutrophils and eosinophils on the top of dermal papillae may form the Piérard micro-abscess, which are typical of this dermatosis, but not pathognomonic. The direct immunofluorescence histology of perilesional skin affected is the gold standard to confirm the diagnosis. It shows the deposition of IgA1 in granular pattern in the lamina lucida of the basement membrane zone. The deposits of IgA in a linear pattern can be found in less than 5% of cases. Indirect immunofluorescence can be used to evaluate the presence of autoantibodies and circulating anti-gliadin, anti-endomysial, anti-reticulin IgA, and anti-epidermal transglutaminase antibodies (anti-tTG) [15]. The first-choice treatment of DH is a strict, life-long GFD which can lead to the resolution of cutaneous and gastrointestinal manifestations with relief in the itching and burning sensation of the vesicle-erythematous-papule.

However, in the first month after the diagnosis or in the inflammatory phases of the disease, in which a GFD alone would not be enough to resolve the cutaneous manifestations, several drugs can be used, including dapsone, steroids or sulfones [10,15].

2.3. Linear IgA Bullous Dermatosis

Linear IgA bullous dermatosis (LABD) is a rare dermatosis characterized by small vesicles and erythematous papules. Pruritus is almost always present with an acute or gradual onset. Up to 24% of the patients affected by LABD also present gluten sensitivity enteropathy and they are responsive to a GFD [16]. LABD and CD often share the same HLA haplotype (i.e., A1, B8, DR3). Although very few case reports have been found in the literature, some authors suggested an association between LABD and gluten sensitivity [16].

3. Urticaria

Urticaria is characterized by intensely pruritic, raised wheals, with or without edema of the deeper cutis. It is usually self-limited, but can be chronic. Chronic urticaria (CU) is defined by recurrent episodes occurring at least twice a week for 6 weeks [17]. The association between CD and CU is widely debated. Ludvigsson and collaborators examined the association between CD and urticaria in 28,900 patients with biopsy-verified CD: 453 patients with CD and no previous diagnosis of urticaria developed urticaria and 79 of these 453 had CU. This confirms that CD is associated with urticaria, especially in its chronic form [17]. CU has been shown to have a genetic association with the human leukocyte antigen HLA-DQ8 alleles. Interestingly, HLAD-Q8 has an association with CD [18]. It has been shown that in CU, there are IgG autoantibodies that inappropriately activate mast cells. The inflammatory response generated in CD probably activates the cells that produce the IgG autoantibodies in CU. It has also been shown that, in patients affected by CD and urticaria, a GFD leads to complete remission of urticaria [19].

4. Hereditary Angioneurotic Edema

Hereditary angioneurotic edema (HANE) is an autosomal dominant genetic disease due to a C1-esterase inhibitor deficiency that leads to an overproduction of bradykinin, causing an increase in vascular permeability. It is characterized by recurrent, marked and diffuse swellings of the subcutaneous and submucosal tissues, painful abdominal attacks, and laryngeal edema with airway obstruction. The symptoms in HANE might be mediated by the activation of the complement system and recent clinical data indicate that the major mediator of angioedema is bradykinin [20]. The therapy consists mainly in the C1-esterase inhibitor concentrate and fresh frozen plasma [20]. The association between CD and hereditary angioneurotic edema, was first reported by Farkas and co-workers [21]. The activation of the pathways of the complement system plays an important role in the pathogenesis of CD and HANE. Gluten ingestion can stimulate complement activity as well as HANE is characterized by an activation of the classic complement pathway [22]. Screening hereditary angioedema patients for CD is warranted if abdominal attacks or neurological symptoms persist despite adequate management. Complement testing is recommended whenever abdominal symptoms persist despite the histological and serological remission of gluten-sensitive enteropathy after the introduction of a GFD [22].

5. Atopic Dermatitis

Atopic dermatitis (AD) is a chronic inflammatory skin disease associated with a heterogeneous group of symptoms and signs. Cutaneous signs and symptoms include erythema, lichenification, prurigo nodules and itch. AD affects 40 million individuals worldwide, and its prevalence is still increasing. Notably, AD appears to be more prevalent among children under five years of age with a decrease in adulthood. The onset of AD occurs primarily in childhood and is thought to precede allergic disorders mediated by IgE sensitization to environmental antigens in the patient affected by atopic triad, as well as AD, asthma, and allergic rhino-conjunctivitis. The complex interaction between genetics, environmental factors, microbiota changes, skin barrier deficiency, immunological derangement, and possibly autoimmunity, contributes to the development of this skin disease [23]. AD has also been linked to CD. Ress and coworkers analyzed the prevalence of CD in children with AD compared with a general pediatric population and showed a four-fold greater risk of developing CD in patients with AD (OR, 4.18; 95% CI, 1.12–15.64). This association may be explained, considering the common cytokine pathways between the two diseases and the screening for CD in patients with AD must be considered in order to prevent the long-term complications of CD [24].

6. Cutaneous Vasculitis

Vasculitis is an inflammatory process affecting the vessel wall and leading to its compromise or destruction with subsequent ischemic and hemorrhagic events. Cutaneous vasculitis is generally characterized by petechiae, palpable purpura and infiltrated erythema indicating dermal superficial, small-vessel vasculitis, or less commonly by nodular erythema, deep ulcers, livedo racemosa, and digital gangrene implicating deep dermal or subcutaneous, muscular-vessel vasculitis [25]. A skin biopsy, extending to subcutis and taken from the earliest, most symptomatic, reddish or purpuric lesion, represents the gold standard for the diagnosis of cutaneous vasculitis. The association between CD and cutaneous vasculitis has been described in several reports [19]. Leukocytoclastic vasculitis (LV), also known as hypersensitivity vasculitis, is a small vessel vasculitis, and it is thought to result from the deposition of circulating immune complexes into the vessel walls, specifically in dermal post-capillary venules, activating the complement pathway. LV is usually limited to the skin and may manifest as palpable purpura, maculopapular rash, bullae, papules, nodules, or ulcers [26]. Meyers et al. reported a case of a young woman, affected by uncontrolled CD, who presented cutaneous LV with the remission of skin lesions after the treatment with a GFD. The coexistence of these two entities might be related to increased intestinal permeability. Exogenous antigens may permeate the damaged CD mucous in larger quantities than normal. This may explain the elevated gluten fraction antibody titer. Moreover, circulating immune complexes are well documented in CD. They probably originate because of the impaired phagocytic function of the reticular endothelium system and subsequently they are deposited in the skin [27,28]. The treatment with a GFD may improve CV lesions in cases associated with CD [28].

7. Erythema Nodosum

Erythema nodosum (EN) is the most common form of panniculitis. It classically presents as tender, warm, erythematous subcutaneous nodules on the bilateral pretibial areas. Although it can occur in both sexes and at any age, it affects predominantly young women [29]. EN associated with CD was reported three times since 1991. It was proposed that the augmented intestinal permeability to various antigens may provoke the skin hypersensitivity reaction [30]. Generally, EN resolves within 8 weeks but as an active disease, it may last up to 18 weeks, and even for a longer period when the antigenic stimulus persists. Furthermore, it has been reported in the literature that CD may coexist with sarcoidosis which is a common cause of EN [31]. EN associated to CD may be far more common than expected. All patients with recurrent or persistent EN of unknown origin should be screened for an underlying CD.

8. Erythema Elevatum Diutinum

Erythema elevatum diutinum (EED) is a rare, chronic and treatable skin condition. The etiology of the disease is unknown, but it has been suggested to be related to high circulating levels of antibodies formed in response to repeated infection. It has many histological mimics and is often associated with several systemic diseases [32]. EED is considered to be a variant of leukocytoclastic vasculitis clinically manifesting as asymptomatic to painful erythematous papules, plaques or nodules, which are usually distributed symmetrically on the extensor surfaces of extremities. It is rarely accompanied by systemic features other than arthritis [32]. Rodriguez-Serna et al. described for the first time, the association between CD and EED in an 11-year-old girl, considering it not a coincidence. With the beginning of the GFD, the cutaneous lesions disappeared and anti-gliadin antibody levels returned to normal. Both conditions have an immune basis in which the increase in IgA appears to play an important role [33]. The pathogenesis of EED is characterized by immune complex deposition, resulting in complement activation, neutrophilic infiltration, and the release of destructive enzymes [32]. Tasanen and others described the presence of granular deposits of IgA and C3 at the derma-epidermal junctions in the affected skin of a patient who presented with EED and CD [34]. Therefore, it is important to evaluate the presence of CD in patients with EED.

9. Necrolytic Migratory Erythema

Necrolytic migratory erythema (NME) is the acronym used for the first time by Wilkinson, to describe the characteristic cutaneous pathology related to glucagonoma. It presents with red-blotch rashes, irregular edges and with vesicles that can be intact or followed by crusting erosions. Frequently, it affects the skin surrounding the lips and upper limbs, more rarely the lower limbs, the abdomen, the groin, the perineum and the buttocks. The affected areas may appear dry or fissured. Initially, the lesion may be exacerbated by pressure or trauma. The phases of lesion development are observed synchronously. Most of the patients have angular cheilitis, stomatitis, glossitis, alopecia, and gastrointestinal symptoms, such as weight loss and diarrhea [35]. NME develops in approximately 70% of patients with glucagonoma syndrome. The etiology is still unclear although a very strong relationship has been noted between hypoaminoacidemia, zinc and a fatty acids deficit due to malabsorption with the severity of NME. A further relationship with NME has been shown in inflammatory autoimmune diseases, such as CD. In fact, the patients affected by CD, who developed the NME, substantially improved the severity of the latter by following a GFD [36].

10. Psoriasis

Psoriasis is a very common chronic inflammatory disease characterized by scaly, well-demarcated, erythematous plaques affecting up to 2% of the general population. The lesions are distributed on different parts of the body, in particular the elbows, knees, trunk, hands and feet [37]. The disease-related quality of life is significantly reduced in patients affected by psoriasis [38]. Psoriatic patients are more likely to have other concomitant autoimmune diseases, such as ulcerative colitis and Crohn disease. CD may be considered as part of these groups. A recent study showed that psoriatic patients have a 2.2-fold risk of being diagnosed with CD compared to healthy controls [39]. A metanalysis showed that IgA AGA, were positive in approximately 14% of psoriatic patients versus 5% of matched controls. Moreover, there was a correlation between the CD antibody positivity and the severity of psoriatic manifestations. Interestingly, the elevated CD antibodies did not always lead to a biopsy-confirmed diagnosis of CD, suggesting that an association between psoriasis and gluten sensitivity, marked by antibody positivity, may be present even in the absence of CD [40]. Psoriasis and CD share different biological mechanisms. Various susceptibility loci are common to both diseases, in particular genes regulating innate and adaptive immune response, such as *RUNX3, TNFAIP3, SOCS1, ELMO1, ETS1, ZMIZ1, UBE2L3.34-36,* and *SH2B3* [41]. Psoriasis and CD have also both been linked to dysregulation in the pathways of Th1, Th17 cells, gamma-delta t-cells and an increased intestinal permeability [42]. Although there are no big clinical trials regarding this argument, a GFD seems to be beneficial for psoriatic patients. Two small clinical trials showed a decrease in serological markers of CD after a GFD and one showed a significant reduction in the psoriasis area severity index. Three case reports also documented the resolution of psoriasis after a GFD [40]. There is also an Italian multicenter study showing that 7 out of 8 patients affected by CD and psoriasis who underwent a GFD showed a significant improvement in the psoriasis area severity index, suggesting a role of gluten in the pathogenesis of both diseases [43].

11. Vitiligo Disease

Vitiligo is an acquired disease characterized by skin depigmentation with the formation of circumscribed white macules, without melanocytes. It predominantly affects the photoexposed areas of the body and the darker phototypes. The disease affects approximately 1% of people in the world and it is often a pathology with inherited characteristics [44]. The etiology is complex and not entirely known. The present dogma suggests that several genetic factors render the melanocyte fragile and susceptible to apoptosis, thus predisposing individuals to developing vitiligo [45]. The association between vitiligo and autoimmune diseases has not yet been fully explained, but genetic data have provided important insights. The susceptibility genes that were identified encode components of the immune system, supporting the hypothesis of a deregulated immune response in vitiligo (HLA class I and II, PTPN22, IL2Rα, GZMB, FOXP3, BACH2, CD80, and CCR6) [46]. The relationship between vitiligo and CD is controversial. The study of Shahmoradi et al. analyzed the frequency of celiac autoantibodies in a group of vitiligo patients compared with the control, involving 128 individuals, 64 vitiligo patients and 64 individuals as the control group [47]. Both IgA EMA and anti-transglutaminase antibodies were measured by the ELISA method in the serum of all participants. The serum of the two vitiligo patients was positive for antibodies. All control groups were seronegative for these antibodies ($p < 0.05$). This study may indicate that both of these autoimmune diseases may be stimulated by a common signal in the immune system that is triggered by a gluten rich diet [47].

12. Behçet's Disease

Behçet's disease (BD) is a chronic-relapsing inflammatory pathology of unknown etiology, characterized by frequent episodes of oral and/or genital ulcers, iritis, associated with various systemic manifestations such as joint, cutaneous and vascular lesions [48]. Behcet's disease can be traced back to an abnormal immune response due to the exposure to a particular antigen in individuals with a genetic predisposition. The onset is between 10 and 30 years with a clear prevalence of the male sex 5–10 times more than women [49]. The stories of oral ulcers and enamel defects have been reported in approximately 25% of patients with CD [50]. There are a few studies in the literature that have elucidated a possible association between BD and CD. Caldas et al. evaluated the association between the two diseases in a 40-year-old woman who presented with asymmetric polyarthralgia, loss of weight, anemia, oral recurrent aphthas (>3/year) and genital ulcerations, inflammatory lower back pain, bowel bleeding and abdominal colic. The biopsy confirmed the diagnosis of CD and a GFD was applied with clinical improvement [51]. Ultimately, it would be desirable for patients with BD to be better investigated for a possible undiagnosed CD.

13. Aphthous Stomatitis

Recurrent aphthous stomatitis (RAS) is a common clinical condition that produces painful ulcerations in the oral cavity. RAS is characterized by multiple recurrent small, round, or ovoid ulcers with circumscribed margins, erythematous haloes typically first presenting in childhood or adolescence. RAS has been recognized for many years as a symptom of CD. A recent meta-analysis showed that celiac patients have greater frequency of RAS (OR = 3.79; 95% CI = 2.67–5.39). RAS patients should be considered at-risk subjects, even in the absence of any gastrointestinal symptoms and should therefore undergo a diagnostic procedure for CD [52]. The etiopathology of RAS is unclear. It is not known whether RAS lesions are directly influenced by the gluten sensitivity disorder, or if they are related to hematinic deficiency with low levels of serum iron, folic acid, and vitamin B12 or trace element deficiencies due to the malabsorption in patients with untreated CD.

14. Oral Lichen Planus

Oral cavity may be involved in CD. The oral manifestations associated to CD are recurrent aphthous stomatitis, glossitis, dental enamel defects, angular cheilitis, burning mouth and oral lichen planus. Oral lichen planus (OLP) is a chronic inflammatory disorder that affects the oral mucosa, gums and tongue with a spectrum of clinical manifestations, including atrophic, erosive, keratotic and ulcerative lesions [53]. OLP, as CD, is characterized by a T-cell autoimmune pathogenesis. Cigic et al. evaluated the prevalence of CD in patients with OLP compared to the controls. In this study, AGA and anti-tTG, were evaluated in 56 OLP patients [54]. CD was diagnosed in eight OLP patients (14.29%) and six OLP patients (10.71%) were positive for IgA Ttg. This confirms the increased frequency of CD in OLP patients [54]. Some erosive, atrophic and ulcerative oral lesions may be caused by underlying haematinic deficiencies associated to the nutrient malabsorption status of CD patients [55].

15. Dermatomyositis

Dermatomyositis (DM) is a rare autoimmune disease that preferentially affects the skin, lungs, muscles and blood vessels and is characterized by proximal and symmetrical muscle weakness with inflammation and damage to the parenchymal cells, causing erythematous and edematous skin manifestations. Usually this is an idiopathic disease. However, it can be associated with other concomitant connective tissue pathologies [56]. It can sometimes occur as a paraneoplastic syndrome associated with gastrointestinal or ovarian malignancies [57]. DM is characterized by the presence of autoantibodies, even if the mechanisms of inflammation and cell damage still remain unclear today [58]. The inflammatory infiltrate in the muscular tissue of DM is represented by T CD4+, B cells and dendritic cells which are preferentially localized around perimysial blood vessels and peripheral areas [59,60]. The inflammation causes damage to the parenchyma and to the blood vessels, so the histological examination shows the presence of a perimysial atrophy, a predominantly perivascular and interfascicular inflammation [59]. The typical histological findings on skin biopsy are vacuolar interface dermatitis with apoptosis, necrotic keratinocytes, and perivascular lymphocytic infiltrate and mucin deposition in the dermis. The inflammatory infiltrate in DM muscle tissue consists of CD4+ T cells, B cells, and dendritic cells that primarily concentrate around perifascicular areas and perimysial blood vessel [58]. Several case reports have highlighted the association between DM and CD [57,61–64].

16. Porphyria

Porphyria, derived from the ancient Greek word "porphura", that is purple, is a group of nine rare diseases: Acute intermittent porphyria (AIP), hereditary coproporphyria (HCP), variegated porphyria (VP), delta-aminolevulinic acid dehydratase deficiency porphyria (ADP), porphyria cutanea tarda (PCT), hepatoerythropoietic porphyria (HEP), congenital erythropoietic porphyria (CEP), erythropoietic protoporphyria (EPP), and X-linked protoporphyria (XLP), characterized by metabolic alterations and caused by malfunctioning of the enzymes involved in the biosynthesis of heme with the accumulation and excretion of porphyrins and their precursors in tissues [65]. The enzyme activity decreases and involves an overproduction of heme precursors, except in XLP [66]. HEP rarely cause clinical manifestations before puberty, as opposed to EPP that manifests symptomatically in the early stages. The precursors of heme of various types accumulate in the liver or bone marrow, which are the most active tissues for the production of heme. All these mechanisms underlie the classification of porphyria as hepatic or erythropoietic. It generally occurs with cutaneous manifestations due to phototoxicity, or with neurological changes such as acute attacks. Based on these differences, the porphyrias are classified as acute or cutaneous. Phototoxicity can occur in all porphyrias, except in ADP and AIP [65]. The urine of patients with this condition may be dark or reddish due to the presence of an excess of porphyrins and related substances. These substances are photosensitizing, and their accumulation causes skin fragility, bullae, scars, hirsutism and the characteristic pigmentation on the photo-exposed areas. This is due both to the release of mediators by leukocytes and mast cells and to the activation of the complement, determining the inflammatory response after photoexposure [67]. Some studies, such as Twaddle and collaborators, have shown a random diagnosis of CD in patients with porphyria [68]. In fact, CD is often associated with DH, underlining some common characteristics of the latter with porphyria. In the VP, the accumulation of 5-aminolevulinic acid and of porfobilinogen provokes both gastrointestinal manifestations and an acute neuropsychiatric syndrome. In this regard, it is important to underline how other works have shown, in patients suffering from CD, a reduction of acute attacks of VP during the GFD [69].

17. Alopecia Areata

Alopecia areata (AA) is a complex, polygenic pathology with autoimmune etiology, which results in the transitory, non-scarring hair loss and the preservation of the hair follicle. By prevalence, it represents the second cause of non-scarring alopecia [70,71]. Clinically, hair loss in alopecia areata manifests itself through very different models. The most frequent pattern is characterized by a small annular or irregular lesion (alopecia areata to patches), usually localized on the scalp, being able to progress until total hair loss, and in this case, the discussion is about total alopecia, associated or not with total loss of all body hair [70]. A biopsy performed on the affected skin shows a lymphocyte infiltrates around the bulb or in the lower part of the hair follicle, thus it suggests an immunological etiology like CD. Recent studies focused on chromosome 6 and more specifically, on the HLA region as the most probable region for the genes that regulate susceptibility to AA [72]. Linkage studies based on a genome-wide association study analysis, have identified an association with many chromosomes and show that AA is a very complex polygenic pathology [70,73]. Both in the AA and in the CD, the presence of organ-specific autoantibodies has been demonstrated [70], with infiltration of T lymphocytes on the lesion site [74]. AA can occur at any age, although most patients develop the disease before the age of 40, with an average age of onset between 25 and 36 years. Early onset between 5 and 10 years, presents itself as a more severe subtype, as an alopecia universalis [75]. Hallaji et al. found that the prevalence of anti-gliadin antibodies in patients with AA had a proportion of 18:100 [76]. In several studies [71,76,77], it has been hypothesized the existence of a CD not diagnosed in patients with AA which improves during a GFD. These positive effects of a GFD on AA, have been associated with the normalization of the immune response [76]. The chronic recurrent phases of CD can be observed during the normal clinical course of AA, and it was noted that patients who followed a GFD regimen showed complete regrowth of hair and other body hair, without highlighting a further recurrence of AA during the follow-up [78]. However, in the study by Mokhtari et al., the frequency distribution of all celiac autoantibodies has been analyzed in patients with AA. The results led to the conclusion that the various biological tests used for the research of subclinical CD do not provide sufficient clear evidence to make the diagnosis of gluten intolerance in patients with AA and other diagnostic approaches are needed [79].

18. Rosacea

Rosacea is an inflammatory skin condition, more frequent in women and primarily characterized by persistent or recurrent episodes of centrofacial erythema [80]. The pathophysiology is not completely understood, but the dysregulation of the immune system as well as changes in the nervous and vascular systems have been identified. Rosacea shares genetic risk loci with autoimmune diseases, such as type 1 diabetes mellitus and CD [81]. One study showed that women with rosacea had a significantly increased risk of CD. In a nationwide cohort study, the prevalence of CD was higher among patients with rosacea when compared to the control subjects (HR = 1.46, 95% CI = 1.11–1.93). However, the pathogenic link is not known. Gastrointestinal symptoms in patients affected by this dermatological condition should warrant clinical suspicion of CD [82].

19. Acquired Hypertrichosis Lanuginosa

Acquired hypertrichosis lanuginose (AHL) is a rare cutaneous manifestation that often underlies the presence of neoplastic pathologies, particularly in the elderly. It is considered as a paraneoplastic manifestation of organic tumor forms, such as a tumor of the gastrointestinal tract, of the lung, of the uterus, of the breast, and often it is indicator of a poor prognosis. It can also be associated with lymphomas. [83]. The etiology is not clear. Corazza and coworkers observed a case of hypertrichosis in a patient suffering from CD [84]. The patient developed a tumor shortly after the diagnosis of CD, confirming that the ACL could represent the unknown tumor spy [84]. However, due to the insufficient data present in the literature, it is not possible to establish a certain correlation.

20. Pyoderma Gangrenosum

Pyoderma gangrenosum (PG) is a rare ulcero-necrotising and neutrophilic dermatosis, whose pathogenesis is unknown. Generally, the main manifestation is a sterile pustule, that rapidly develops into a painful ulcer from the erythematous border [85]. The diagnosis is often a challenge for the clinician and it is often achieved by exclusion. In the literature, many studies have shown the association between inflammatory bowel diseases and in particular, Crohn's disease and ulcerative colitis, and skin manifestations including PG [86]. Weizman et al. have described one of the largest case series of PG among patients with inflammatory bowel disease (IBD) [87]. Moreover, it was observed that the female sex and young age at diagnosis of IBD are predictive factors involved in the development of main cutaneous manifestations [88]. Furthermore, refractory CD resistant to steroids and immunosuppressive drugs has been reported to be associated to PG [89]. The appearance of a pustule transforming to an ulcer in a patient with CD should always arise the suspect for PG [87].

21. Ichthyosiform Dermatoses

Ichthyosiform dermatoses are a group of a skin disorders characterized by clinically evident thickening of the stratum corneum, dry skin and often erythroderma. The term ichthyosis derives from the Greek "ichthys" that means fish, referring to the cutaneous scaling characteristic of these disorders, which is said to resemble the scales of a fish. The attention for this pathology is quite recent. In fact, the first international ichthyosis conference classification was approved in 2009 [90]. The first case report associating the ichthyosis with CD was observed by Menni and co-workers. They reported the clinical history of a twenty-nine year-old woman, who presented ichthyosiform skin manifestations [91]. After just over 10 years, another case that showed this association was reported. In this case, the patient was younger than the first case, but also affected by osteoporosis and secondary hyperparathyroidism. Although the GFD did not allow a complete disappearance of the cutaneous manifestations, it favored an improvement in the quality of life [92].

22. Pellagra

Pellagra is a rare disease caused by niacin deficiency and characterized by a classical triad: Dermatitis, dementia and diarrhea, known as "3D" [93]. The skin signs are the first to appear in over 80% of cases. Initially, itchy and erythematous lesions appear on the area of photo-exposed skin and generally, they are bilateral and symmetrical lesions localized on the dorsum of the hands, arms, face and neck. Subsequently, the gastrointestinal and neurological symptoms occur [93]. In 1937, a case was published of a 15-month-old child with skin manifestations compatible with a non-classical form of pellagra and the simultaneous presence of gastrointestinal disorders related to CD [94]. More than 60 years later, Schattner described another case of a 70-years-old man with a pellagra-like syndrome due to CD [95]. No other cases have been reported, determining a weak association between the two conditions.

23. Generalized Acquired Cutis Laxa

Cutis laxa (CL), also called elastolysis or dermatomegaly, includes a heterogenous group of disorders that affects the elastic tissue and it is characterized by the presence of loose and redundant skin, caused by a reduced number and abnormal properties of elastic fibers in the derma [96]. The etiopathogenesis is still not fully known; it can be congenital or acquired [97]. Only one case in the literature shows the coexistence of acquired CL and CD. In this case, the clinical suspicion of CL was confirmed histologically and analyzed through direct immunofluorescence. The latter has highlighted the presence of IgA deposits in the papillary dermis. It is possible to hypothesize that the IgA deposit constitutes the base of the pathophysiological link between the two diseases [71,98].

24. Skin Malignancies

The variations of the incidence of the skin malignancies in patients affected by CD is a very interesting topic. A study by Ilus et al. studied a population of 32,439 adult celiac patients to evaluate the relative risk for each kind of malignancies [99]. Among cutaneous cancer, a major incidence was registered for basal cell carcinoma and a slightly minor incidence for melanoma [99]. There is instead a known association between CD and lymphomas [99], and cutaneous lymphomas seem also associated to CD. Various case reports show this association, the last one being reported in 2016. The association of cutaneous lymphoma with CD may be determined by a lymphocytic stimulation carried out by the presence of a constant antigen, such as gluten, in the gastrointestinal tract. Some researchers [100] suggested that in predisposed individuals, the resulting dysplastic T cells may migrate into cutis, causing cutaneous T cell lymphoma. The adherence to a GFD decreases the risk for malignancy.

25. Conclusions

CD is an autoimmune enteropathy associated with several extra-intestinal diseases, including various skin manifestations. Different hypotheses have been proposed to explain the possible mechanisms involved in every association between CD and cutaneous manifestations. An abnormal small intestinal permeability seems to be implicated in various dermatological manifestations. The inability of the small intestine to operate as a barrier may allow a major penetration of exogenous antigens with a consequent immunological response that leads to vascular alterations and to malabsorption with secondary vitamin and amino acidic deficiency. However, on the basis of the revision of the literature by the levels of evidence, it can be concluded that only a few associations are very strong and in particular, DH and psoriasis. The other associations between CD and skin diseases are based on case-reports and case series, with very few multicentric controlled studies. In this way, to better assess the involvement of the cutaneous district in CD, large multicentric controlled studies are required. Nevertheless, screening for CD in patients suffering from chronic cutaneous diseases seems to be justified considering that a GFD can significantly improve both gastrointestinal and systemic symptoms.

Author Contributions: Conceptualization, L.A.; methodology, L.A., S.D. and L.B. (Luigi Bennardo); resources, L.B. (Luigi Bennardo), M.P. and M.S.; data curation, S.D.; writing—original draft preparation, L.A. and L.B. (Luigi Boccuto); writing—review and editing L.A., S.D., I.P. and L.B. (Luigi Bennardo); visualization, F.L. and C.P.; supervision, S.P.N.

Funding: This research received no external funding.

Conflicts of Interest: The authors declare no conflicts of interest.

References

1. Lebwohl, B.; Sanders, D.S.; Green, P.H.R. Coeliac disease. *Lancet* **2018**, *391*, 70–81. [CrossRef]
2. Leonard, M.M.; Sapone, A.; Catassi, C.; Fasano, A. Celiac disease and nonceliac gluten sensitivity: A review. *JAMA* **2017**, *318*, 647–656. [CrossRef] [PubMed]
3. Abenavoli, L.; Proietti, I.; Zaccone, V. Celiac disease: From gluten to skin. *Expert. Rev. Clin. Immunol.* **2009**, *5*, 789–800. [CrossRef] [PubMed]
4. Abenavoli, L.; Proietti, I.; Leggio, L. Cutaneous manifestations in celiac disease. *World J. Gastroenterol.* **2006**, *12*, 843–852. [CrossRef]
5. Hujoel, I.A.; Reilly, N.R.; Rubio-Tapia, A. Celiac disease: Clinical features and diagnosis. *Gastroenterol. Clin. North Am.* **2019**, *48*, 19–37. [CrossRef] [PubMed]
6. OCEBM Levels of Evidence. Available online: https://www.cebm.net/?o=1025 (accessed on 31 May 2019).
7. Palleria, C.; Bennardo, L.; Dastoli, S.; Iannone, L.F.; Silvestri, M.; Manti, A.; Nisticò, S.P.; Russo, E.; De Sarro, G. Angiotensin-converting-enzyme inhibitors and angiotensin II receptor blockers induced pemphigus: A case series and literature review. *Dermatol. Ther.* **2018**, *32*, e12748. [CrossRef]
8. Labidi, A.; Serghini, M.; Karoui, S.; Ben Mustapha, N.; Boubaker, J.; Filali, A. Epilepsy, pemphigus and celiac disease: An exceptional association. *Tunis Med.* **2014**, *92*, 585–586.
9. Drago, F.; Cacciapuoti, M.; Basso, M.; Parodi, A.; Rebora, A. Pemphigus improving with gluten-free diet. *Acta Derm. Venereol.* **2005**, *85*, 84–85. [CrossRef]
10. Antiga, E.; Caproni, M. The diagnosis and treatment of dermatitis herpetiformis. *Clin. Cosmet. Investig. Dermatol.* **2015**, *13*, 257–265. [CrossRef]

11. Salmi, T.T.; Hervonen, K.; Kurppa, K.; Collin, P.; Kaukinen, K.; Reunala, T. Celiac disease evolving into dermatitis herpetiformis in patients adhering to normal or gluten-free diet. *Scand. J. Gastroenterol.* **2015**, *50*, 387–392. [CrossRef]
12. Hull, C.M.; Liddle, M.; Hansen, N. Elevation of IgA anti-epidermal transglutaminase antibodies in dermatitis herpetiformis. *Br. J. Dermatol.* **2008**, *159*, 120–124. [CrossRef] [PubMed]
13. Reunala, T.; Salmi, T.T.; Hervonen, K.; Kaukinen, K.; Collin, P. Dermatitis herpetiformis: A common extraintestinal manifestation of coeliac disease. *Nutrients* **2018**, *12*, 10. [CrossRef] [PubMed]
14. Husby, S.; Koletzko, S.; Korponay-Szabó, I.R.; Mearin, M.L.; Phillips, A.; Shamir, R.; Troncone, R.; Giersiepen, K.; Branski, D.; Catassi, C.; et al. European society for pediatric gastroenterology, hepatology, and nutrition guidelines for the diagnosis of coeliac disease. *J. Pediatr. Gastroenterol. Nutr.* **2012**, *54*, 136–160. [CrossRef] [PubMed]
15. Mendes, F.B.; Hissa-Elian, A.; Abreu, M.A.; Gonçalves, V.S. Review: Dermatitis herpetiformis. *Ann. Bras. Dermatol.* **2013**, *88*, 594–599. [CrossRef] [PubMed]
16. Egan, C.A.; Smith, E.P.; Taylor, T.B.; Meyer, L.J.; Samowitz, W.S.; Zone, J.J. Linear IgA bullous dermatosis responsive to a gluten-free diet. *Am. J. Gastroenterol.* **2001**, *96*, 1927–1929. [CrossRef] [PubMed]
17. Ludvigsson, J.F.; Lindelöf, B.; Rashtak, S.; Rubio-Tapia, A.; Murray, J.A. Does urticaria risk increase in patients with celiac disease? A large population-based cohort study. *Eur. J. Dermatol.* **2013**, *23*, 681–687. [CrossRef] [PubMed]
18. O'Donnell, B.; O'Neill, C.; Francis, D.; Niimi, N.; Barr, R.; Barlow, R.; Kobza, B.A.; Welsh, K.; Greaves, M. Human leucocyte antigen class II associations in chronic idiopathic urticaria. *Br. J. Dermatol.* **1999**, *140*, 853–858. [CrossRef] [PubMed]
19. Rodrigo, L.; Beteta-Gorriti, V.; Alvarez, N.; De Castro, C.G.; De Dios, A.; Palacios, L.; Santos-Juanes, J. Cutaneous and mucosal manifestations associated with celiac disease. *Nutrients* **2018**, *21*, 10. [CrossRef] [PubMed]
20. Davis, A.E., 3rd. Oedema: A current state-of-the-art review, III: Mechanisms of hereditary angioedema. *Ann. Allergy Asthma Immunol.* **2008**, *100*, S7–S12. [CrossRef]
21. Farkas, H.; Visy, B.; Fekete, B.; Karádi, I.; Kovács, J.B.; Kovács, I.B.; Kalmár, L.; Tordai, A.; Varga, L. Association of celiac disease and hereditary angioneurotic edema. *Am. J. Gastroenterol.* **2002**, *97*, 2682–2683. [CrossRef]
22. Henao, M.P.; Kraschnewski, J.L.; Kelbel, T.; Craig, T.J. Diagnosis and screening of patients with hereditary angioedema in primary care. *Ther. Clin. Risk Manag.* **2016**, *12*, 701–711. [CrossRef] [PubMed]
23. Boothe, D.W.; Tarbox, J.A.; Tarbox, M.B. Atopic dermatitis: Pathophysiology. *Adv. Exp. Med. Biol.* **2017**, *1027*, 21–37.
24. Ress, K.; Annus, T.; Putnik, U.; Luts, K.; Uibo, R.; Uibo, O. Celiac disease in children with atopic dermatitis. *Pediatr. Dermatol.* **2014**, *31*, 483–488. [CrossRef] [PubMed]
25. Chen, K.R.; Carlson, J.A. Clinical approach to cutaneous vasculitis. *Am. J. Clin. Dermatol.* **2008**, *9*, 71–92. [CrossRef] [PubMed]
26. Baigrie, D.; Crane, J.S. *Leukocytoclastic Vasculitis (Hypersensitivity Vasculitis)*; StatPearls Publishing: Treasure Island, FL, USA, 2018.
27. Meyers, S.; Dikman, S.; Spiera, H.; Schultz, N.; Janowitz, H. Cutaneous vasculitis complicating coeliac disease. *Gut* **1981**, *22*, 61–64. [CrossRef] [PubMed]
28. Caproni, M.; Bonciolini, V.; D'Errico, A.; Antiga, E.; Fabbri, P. Celiac disease and dermatologic manifestations: Many skin clue to unfold gluten-sensitive enteropathy. *Gastroenterol. Res. Pract.* **2012**, *2012*, 952753. [CrossRef]
29. Spagnuolo, R.; Dastoli, S.; Silvestri, M. Anti interleukin 12/23 in the treatment of erythema nodosum and Crohn disease: A case report. *Dermatol. Ther.* **2019**, *32*, e12811. [CrossRef]
30. Fretzayas, A.; Moustaki, M.; Liapi, O.; Nicolaidou, P. Erythema nodosum in a child with celiac disease. *Case Rep. Pediatr.* **2011**, *2011*, 935153. [CrossRef]
31. Papadopoulos, K.I.; Sjoberg, K.; Lindgren, S.; Hallengren, B. Evidence of gastrointestinal immunoreactivity in patients with sarcoidosis. *J. Int. Med.* **1999**, *245*, 525–531. [CrossRef]
32. Momen, S.E.; Jorizzo, J.; Al-Niaimi, F. Erythema elevatum diutinum: A review of presentation and treatment. *J. Eur. Acad. Dermatol. Venereol.* **2014**, *28*, 1594–1602. [CrossRef]

33. Rodriguez-Serna, M.; Fortea, J.M.; Perez, A.; Febrer, I.; Ribes, C.; Aliaga, A. Erythema elevatum diutinum associated with celiac disease: Response to a gluten-free diet. *Pediatr. Dermatol.* **1993**, *10*, 125–128. [CrossRef] [PubMed]
34. Tasanen, K.; Raudasoja, R.; Kallioinen, M.; Ranki, A. Erythema elevatum diutinum in association with coeliac disease. *Br. J. Dermatol.* **1997**, *136*, 624–627. [CrossRef] [PubMed]
35. Compton, N.L.; Chien, A.J. A rare but revealing sign: Necrolytic migratory erythema. *Am. J. Med.* **2013**, *126*, 387–389. [CrossRef]
36. Tamura, A.; Ogasawara, T.; Fujii, Y.; Kanek, H.; Nakayama, A.; Higuchi, S.; Hashimoto, N.; Miyabayashi, Y.; Fujimoto, M.; Komai, E. Glucagonoma with necrolytic migratory erythema: Metabolic profile and detection of biallelic inactivation of DAXX gene. *J. Clin. Endocrinol. Metab.* **2018**, *103*, 2417–2423. [CrossRef] [PubMed]
37. Bennardo, L.; Del Duca, E.; Dastoli, S.; Schipani, G.; Scali, E.; Silvestri, M.; Nisticò, S.P. Potential applications of topical oxygen therapy in dermatology. *Dermatol. Pract. Concept.* **2018**, *8*, 272–276. [CrossRef] [PubMed]
38. Dattola, A.; Silvestri, M.; Bennardo, L.; Del Duca, E.; Longo, C.; Bianchi, L.; Nisticò, S.P. Update of calcineurin inhibitors to treat inverse psoriasis: A systematic review. *Dermatol. Ther.* **2018**, *31*, e12728. [CrossRef] [PubMed]
39. Wu, J.J.; Nguyen, T.U.; Poon, K.Y.; Herrinton, L.J. The association of psoriasis with autoimmune diseases. *J. Am. Acad. Dermatol.* **2012**, *67*, 924–930. [CrossRef]
40. Bhatia, B.K.; Millsop, J.W.; Debbaneh, M.; Koo, J.; Linos, E.; Liao, W. Diet and psoriasis, part II: Celiac disease and role of a gluten-free diet. *J. Am. Acad. Dermatol.* **2014**, *71*, 350–358. [CrossRef]
41. Tsoi, L.C.; Spain, S.L.; Knight, J.; Ellinghaus, E.; Stuart, P.E.; Capon, F.; Ding, J.; Li, Y.; Tejasvi, T.; Gudjonsson, J.E.; et al. Identification of 15 new psoriasis susceptibility loci highlights the role of innate immunity. *Nat. Genet.* **2012**, *44*, 1341–1348. [CrossRef]
42. Cianci, R.; Cammarota, G.; Frisullo, G.; Pagliari, D.; Ianiro, G.; Martini, M.; Frosali, S.; Plantone, D.; Damato, V.; Casciano, F.; et al. Tissue-infiltrating lymphocytes analysis reveals large modifications of the duodenal "immunological niche" in coeliac disease after gluten-free diet. *Clin. Transl. Gastroenterol.* **2012**, *3*, e28. [CrossRef]
43. De Bastiani, R.; Gabrielli, M.; Lora, L.; Napoli, L.; Tosetti, C.; Pirrotta, E. Association between coeliac disease and psoriasis: Italian primary care multicentre study. *Dermatology* **2015**, *230*, 156–160. [CrossRef] [PubMed]
44. Magna, P.; Elbuluk, N.; Orlow, S.J. Recent advances in understanding vitiligo. *F1000Research* **2016**, *5*, pii:F1000 Faculty Rev-2234.
45. Boissy, R.E.; Manga, P. On the etiology of contact/occupational vitiligo. *Pigment Cell Res.* **2004**, *17*, 208–214. [CrossRef] [PubMed]
46. Ezzedine, K.; Lim, H.W.; Suzuki, T.; Katayama, I.; Hamzavi, I.; Lan, C.C.; Goh, B.K.; Anbar, T.; De Castro, S.C.; Lee, A.Y. Revised classification/nomenclature of vitiligo and related issues: The Vitiligo Global Issues Consensus Conference. *Pigment Cell Melanoma Res.* **2012**, *25*, E1–E13. [CrossRef] [PubMed]
47. Shahmoradi, Z.; Najafian, J.; Naeini, F.F.; Fahimipour, F. Vitiligo and autoantibodies of celiac disease. *Int. J. Prev. Med.* **2013**, *4*, 200–203. [PubMed]
48. Abenavoli, L. Behçet's disease and celiac disease: A rare association or a possible link? *Rheumatol. Int.* **2010**, *30*, 1405–1406. [CrossRef] [PubMed]
49. Abenavoli, L.; Proietti, I.; Vonghia, L.; Leggio, L.; Ferrulli, A.; Capizzi, R.; Mirijello, A.; Cardone, S.; Malandrino, N.; Leso, V.; et al. Intestinal malabsorption and skin diseases. *Dig. Dis.* **2008**, *26*, 167–174. [CrossRef] [PubMed]
50. Cheng, J.; Malahias, T.; Brar, P.; Minaya, M.T.; Green, P.H. The association between celiac disease, dental enamel defects, and aphthous ulcers in a United States cohort. *J. Clin. Gastroenterol.* **2010**, *44*, 191–194. [CrossRef] [PubMed]
51. Caldas, C.A.M.; Verderame, L.L.; De Carvalho, J.F. Behçet's disease associated with celiac disease: A very rare association. *Rheumatol. Int.* **2010**, *30*, 523–525. [CrossRef] [PubMed]
52. Nieri, M.; Tofani, E.; Defraia, E.; Giuntini, V.; Franchi, L. Enamel defects and aphthous stomatitis in celiac and healthy subjects: Systematic review and meta-analysis of controlled studies. *J. Dent.* **2017**, *65*, 1–10. [CrossRef] [PubMed]

53. Pastore, L.; Carroccio, A.; Compilato, D.; Panzarella, V.; Serpico, R.; Lo Muzio, L. Oral manifestations of celiac disease. *J. Clin. Gastroenterol.* **2008**, *42*, 224–232. [CrossRef] [PubMed]
54. Cigic, L.; Gavic, L.; Simunic, M.; Ardalic, Z.; Biocina-Lukenda, D. Increased prevalence of celiac disease in patients with oral lichen planus. *Clin. Oral Investig.* **2015**, *19*, 627–635. [CrossRef] [PubMed]
55. Compilato, D.; Carroccio, A.; Campisi, G. Hidden coeliac disease in patients suffering from oral lichen planus. *J. Eur. Acad. Dermatol. Venereol.* **2012**, *26*, 390–391. [CrossRef] [PubMed]
56. Fernandez, A.P. Connective tissue disease: Current Concepts. *Dermatol. Clin.* **2019**, *37*, 37–48. [CrossRef] [PubMed]
57. Song, M.S.; Farber, D.; Bitton, A.; Jass, J.; Singer, M.; Karpati, G. Dermatomyositis associated with celiac disease: Response to a gluten-free diet. *Can. J. Gastroenterol.* **2006**, *20*, 433–435. [CrossRef] [PubMed]
58. Kao, L.; Chung, L.; Fiorentino, D.F. Pathogenesis of dermatomyositis: Role of cytokines and interferon. *Curr. Rheumatol. Rep.* **2011**, *13*, 225–232. [CrossRef] [PubMed]
59. Dalakas, M.C.; Hohlfeld, R. Polymyositis and dermatomyositis. *Lancet* **2003**, *362*, 971–982. [CrossRef]
60. Caproni, M.; Torchia, D.; Cardinali, C.; Volpi, W.; Del Bianco, E.; D'Agata, A.; Fabbri, P. Infiltrating cells, related cytokines and chemokine receptors in lesional skin of patients with dermatomyositis. *Br. J. Dermatol.* **2004**, *151*, 784–791. [CrossRef] [PubMed]
61. De Paepe, B.; Creus, K.K.; De Bleecker, J.L. Role of cytokines and chemokines in idiopathic inflammatory myopathies. *Curr. Opin. Rheumatol.* **2009**, *21*, 610–616. [CrossRef]
62. Molnár, K.; Torma, K.; Siklós, K.; Csanády, K.; Korponay-Szabó, I.; Szalai, Z. Juvenile dermatomyositis and celiac disease. A rare association. *Eur. J. Pediatr. Dermatol.* **2006**, *16*, 153–157.
63. Marie, I.; Lecomte, F.; Hachulla, E. An uncommon association: Celiac disease and dermatomyositis in adults. *Clin. Exp. Rheumatol.* **2001**, *19*, 201–203. [PubMed]
64. Iannone, F.; Lapadula, G. Dermatomyositis and celiac disease association: A further case. *Clin. Exp. Rheumatol.* **2001**, *19*, 757–758. [PubMed]
65. Ramanujam, V.M.; Anderson, K.E. Porphyria diagnostics-part 1: A brief overview of the porphyrias. *Curr. Protoc. Hum. Genet.* **2015**, *86*, 1–26.
66. Ducamp, S.; Schneider-Yin, X.; De Rooij, F.; Clayton, J.; Fratz, E.J.; Rudd, A.; Ostapowicz, G.; Varigos, G.; Lefebvre, T.; Deybach, J.C.; et al. Molecular and functional analysis of the C-terminal region of human erythroid-specific 5-aminolevulinic synthase associated with X-linked dominant protoporphyria (XLDPP). *Hum. Mol. Genet.* **2013**, *22*, 1280–1288. [CrossRef]
67. Anderson, K.E. *Handbook of Porphyrin Science with Applications in Chemistry, Physics, Materials Science, Engineering, Biology, and Medicine, Vol. 29: Porphyrias and Sideroblastic Anemias*; World Scientific Publishing Co.: Hackensack, NJ, USA, 2014; pp. 370–406.
68. Twaddle, S.; Wassif, W.S.; Deacon, A.C.; Peters, T.J. Celiac disease in patients with variegate porphyria. *Dig. Dis. Sci.* **2001**, *46*, 1506–1508. [CrossRef] [PubMed]
69. Urban-Kowalczyk, M.; Œmigielski, J.; Gmitrowicz, A. Neuropsychiatric symptoms and celiac disease. *Neuropsychiatr. Dis. Treat.* **2014**, *10*, 1961–1964. [CrossRef] [PubMed]
70. Pratt, H.; King, L.; Messenger, A.; Christiano, A.; Sundberg, J. Alopecia areata. *Nat. Rev. Dis. Primers.* **2017**, *3*, 17011. [CrossRef] [PubMed]
71. Hietikko, M.; Hervonen, K.; Salmi, T.; Ilus, T.; Zone, J.J.; Kaukinen, K.; Reunala, T.; Lindfors, K. Disappearance of epidermal transglutaminase and IgA deposits from the papillary dermis of patients with dermatitis herpetiformis after a long-term gluten-free diet. *Br. J. Dermatol.* **2018**, *178*, e198–e201. [CrossRef] [PubMed]
72. Barahmani, N.; De Andrade, M.; Slusser, J.P.; Wei, Q.; Hordinsky, M.; Prezzo, V.H.; Christiano, A.; Norris, D.; Reveille, J.; Duvic, M. Human leukocyte antigen class II alleles are associated with risk of alopecia areata. *J. Invest. Dermatol.* **2008**, *128*, 240–243. [CrossRef]
73. Betz, R.C.; Petukhova, L.; Ripke, S. Genome-wide meta-analysis in alopecia areata resolves HLA associations and reveals two new susceptibility loci. *Nature Commun.* **2015**, *6*, 5966. [CrossRef]
74. Carroll, J.; McElwee, K.J.; King, L.E.; Byrne, M.C.; Sundberg, J.P. Gene array profiling and immunomodulation studies define a cell mediated immune response underlying the pathogenesis of alopecia areata in a mouse model and humans. *J. Invest. Dermatol.* **2002**, *119*, 392–402. [CrossRef] [PubMed]

75. Fricke, A.C.V.; Miteva, M. Epidemiology and burden of alopecia areata: A systematic review. *Clin. Cosmet. Investig. Dermatol.* **2015**, *8*, 397–403.
76. Hallaji, Z.; Akhyani, M.; Ehsani, A.H.; Noormohammadpour, P.; Gholamali, F.; Bagheri, M.; Jahromi, J. Prevalence of anti-gliadin antibody in patients with alopecia areata: A case-control study. *Tehran Univ. Med. J.* **2011**, *68*, 738–742.
77. Collin, P.; Reunala, T. Recognition and management of the cutaneous manifestations of Celiac disease. *Am J. Clin. Dermatol.* **2003**, *4*, 13–20. [CrossRef]
78. Naveh, Y.; Rosenthal, E.; Ben-Arieh, Y.; Etzioni, A. Celiac disease-associated alopecia in childhood. *J. Pediatr.* **1999**, *134*, 362–364. [CrossRef]
79. Mokhtari, F.; Panjehpour, T.; Naeini, F.; Hosseini, S.; Nilforoushzadeh, M.; Matin, M. The frequency distribution of celiac autoantibodies in alopecia areata. *Int. J Prev. Med.* **2016**, *7*, 109. [CrossRef] [PubMed]
80. Van Zuuren, E.J. Rosacea. *Nat. Engl. J. Med.* **2017**, *377*, 1754–1764. [CrossRef] [PubMed]
81. Chang, A.L.S.; Raber, I.; Xu, J.; Li, R.; Spitale, R.; Chen, J.; Kiefer, A.K.; Tian, C.; Eriksson, N.K.; Hinds, D.A.; et al. Assessment of the genetic basis of rosacea by genome-wide association study. *J. Invest. Dermatol.* **2015**, *135*, 1548–1555. [CrossRef]
82. Egeberg, A.; Weinstock, L.B.; Thyssen, E.P.; Gislason, G.H.; Thyssen, J.P. Rosacea and gastrointestinal disorders: A population-based cohort study. *Br. J. Dermatol.* **2017**, *176*, 100–106. [CrossRef]
83. Sánchez-Estella, J.; Yuste, M.; Santos, J.C.; Alonso, M.T. Acquired paraneoplastic hypertrichosis lanuginose. *Actas Dermosifiliogr.* **2005**, *96*, 459–461. [CrossRef]
84. Corazza, G.R.; Masina, M.; Passarini, B.; Neri, I.; Varotti, C. Ipertricosi lanuginosa acquisita associata a sindrome celiaca. *G. Ital. Dermatol. Venereol.* **1988**, *123*, 611–612. [PubMed]
85. Braswell, S.F.; Kostopoulos, T.C.; Ortega-Loayza, A.G. Pathophysiology of pyoderma gangrenosum (PG): An updated review. *J. Am. Acad. Dermatol.* **2015**, *73*, 691–698. [CrossRef] [PubMed]
86. Hindryckx, P.; Novak, G.; Costanzo, A.; Danese, S. Disease-related and drug-induced skin manifestations in inflammatory bowel disease. *Expert Rev. Gastroenterol. Hepatol.* **2017**, *11*, 203–214. [CrossRef] [PubMed]
87. Weizman, A.V.; Huang, B.; Targan, S.; Dubinsky, M.; Fleshner, P.; Kaur, M.; Ippoliti, A.; Panikkath, D.; Vasiliauskas, E.; Shih, D.; et al. Pyoderma gangrenosum among patients with inflammatory bowel disease: A descriptive cohort study. *J. Cutan. Med. Surg.* **2014**, *19*, 125–131. [CrossRef] [PubMed]
88. Ampuero, J.; Rojas-Feria, M.; Castro-Fernández, M.; Cano, C.; Romero-Gómez, M. Predictive factors for erythema nodosum and pyoderma gangrenosum in inflammatory bowel disease. *J. Gastroenterol. Hepatol.* **2014**, *29*, 291–295. [CrossRef] [PubMed]
89. Sedda, S.; Caruso, R.; Marafini, I. Pyoderma gangrenosum in refractory celiac disease: A case report. *BMC Gastroenterol.* **2013**, *13*, 162. [CrossRef] [PubMed]
90. Oji, V. Clinical presentation and etiology of ichthyoses. Overview of the new nomenclature and classification. *Hautarzt* **2010**, *61*, 891–902. [CrossRef] [PubMed]
91. Menni, S.; Boccardi, D.; Brusasco, A. Ichthyosis revealing coeliac disease. *Eur. J. Dermatol.* **2000**, *10*, 398–399.
92. Nenna, R.; D'Eufemia, P.; Celli, M.; Mennini, M.; Petrarca, L.; Zambrano, A.; Montuori, M.; La Pietra, M.; Bonamico, M. Celiac disease and lamellar ichthyosis. Case study analysis and review of the literature. *Acta Dermatovenerol. Croat.* **2011**, *19*, 268–270.
93. De Oliveira, A.A.; Bortolato, T.; Bernardes, F.F. Pellagra. *J. Emerg. Med.* **2018**, *54*, 238–240. [CrossRef]
94. Lightwood, R.; Smallpeice, V. Coeliac disease with a conditioned vitamin deficiency resembling, but not typical of Pellagra. *Proc. R. Soc. Med.* **1937**, *31*, 71–73. [CrossRef] [PubMed]
95. Schattner, A. 70-year-old man with isolated weight loss and a pellagra-like syndrome due to celiac disease. *Yale J. Biol. Med.* **1999**, *72*, 15–18. [PubMed]
96. Paulsen, I.F.; Bredgaard, R.; Hesse, B.; Steiniche, T.; Henriksen, T.F. Acquired cutis laxa: Diagnostic and therapeutic considerations. *J. Plast. Reconstr. Aesthet. Surg.* **2014**, *67*, e242–e243. [CrossRef] [PubMed]
97. Berk, D.R.; Bentley, D.D.; Bayliss, S.J.; Lind, A.; Urban, Z. Cutis laxa: A review. *J. Am. Acad. Dermatol.* **2012**, *66*, 842-e1–842-e17. [CrossRef] [PubMed]
98. García-Patos, V.; Pujol, R.M.; Barnadas, M.A.; Pérez, M.; Moreno, A.; Condomines, J.; Gelpi, C.; Rodríguez, J.L.; De Moragas, J.M. Generalized acquired cutis laxa ssociated with coeliac disease: Evidence of immunoglobulin A deposits on the dermal elastic fibers. *Br. J. Dermatol.* **1996**, *135*, 130–134. [CrossRef] [PubMed]

99. Ilus, T.; Kaukinen, K.; Virta, L.J.; Pukkala, E.; Collin, P. Incidence of malignancies in diagnosed celiac patients: A population-based estimate. *Am. J. Gastroenterol.* **2014**, *109*, 1471–1477. [CrossRef] [PubMed]
100. Porter, W.M.; Dawe, S.A.; Bunker, C.B. Dermatitis herpetiformis and cutaneous T-cell lymphoma. *Clin. Exp. Dermatol.* **2001**, *26*, 304–305. [CrossRef] [PubMed]

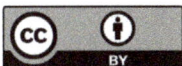

© 2019 by the authors. Licensee MDPI, Basel, Switzerland. This article is an open access article distributed under the terms and conditions of the Creative Commons Attribution (CC BY) license (http://creativecommons.org/licenses/by/4.0/).

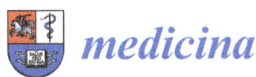

Review

Hematologic Manifestations in Celiac Disease—A Practical Review

Daniel Vasile Balaban [1,2,*], Alina Popp [1,3,4], Florentina Ionita Radu [2,5] and Mariana Jinga [1,2]

1. "Carol Davila" University of Medicine and Pharmacy, 020021 Bucharest, Romania
2. Gastroenterology Department, "Dr. Carol Davila" Central Military Emergency University Hospital, 010825 Bucharest, Romania
3. Pediatrics Department, "Alessandrescu-Rusescu" National Institute for Mother and Child Health, 020395 Bucharest, Romania
4. Faculty of Medicine and Health Technology, Tampere University and Tampere University Hospital, 33100 Tampere, Finland
5. Faculty of Medicine, Titu Maiorescu University, 004051 Bucharest, Romania
* Correspondence: vasile.balaban@umfcd.ro

Received: 7 May 2019; Accepted: 8 July 2019; Published: 15 July 2019

Abstract: Celiac disease (CD) is a systemic autoimmune disease driven by gluten-ingestion in genetically predisposed individuals. Although it primarily affects the small bowel, CD can also involve other organs and manifest as an extraintestinal disease. Among the extraintestinal features of CD, hematologic ones are rather frequent and consist of anemia, thrombocytosis (thrombocytopenia also, but rare), thrombotic or hemorrhagic events, IgA deficiency, hyposplenism, and lymphoma. These hematologic alterations can be the sole manifestation of the disease and should prompt for CD testing in a suggestive clinical scenario. Recognition of these atypical, extraintestinal presentations, including hematologic ones, could represent a great opportunity to increase the diagnostic rate of CD, which is currently one of the most underdiagnosed chronic digestive disorders worldwide. In this review, we summarize recent evidence regarding the hematological manifestations of CD, with focus on practical recommendations for clinicians.

Keywords: celiac disease; anemia; lymphoma; IgA deficiency

1. Introduction

Celiac disease (CD) is a chronic, autoimmune condition triggered by gluten ingestion in genetically susceptible individuals. It can develop at any time throughout the life of individuals carrying the predisposing DQ2/DQ8 haplotype, leading to a gluten-dependent small-bowel inflammation consisting of villous atrophy and crypt hyperplasia. As gluten is the culprit in driving the autoimmune-mediated villous atrophy, its removal from the diet of CD patients leads to symptom relief, restoring of small bowel mucosa, and avoidance of complications. CD has an overall prevalence of about 1% worldwide, with higher rates reported in Northern European countries [1,2].

CD is nowadays widely recognized as a systemic disorder and not only a disease of the small bowel, as many of the adults diagnosed with CD present with extraintestinal manifestations. In fact, the typical presentation with malabsorption syndrome is seen mostly in children and quite rare in adults, who often present with mild, intermittent, and low-intensity digestive symptoms and a wide spectrum of extraintestinal manifestations [3–6].

The extraintestinal features of CD include a wide range of rheumatologic, neurologic, hematologic, endocrine, metabolic, and dermatologic manifestations [6–9]. Among them, hematologic findings are one of the most frequent presentations, and sometimes, they can represent the sole manifestation of the disease [10]. In this setting, a high index of suspicion for CD is needed in patients with unexplained, isolated hematological abnormalities, and this depends on better awareness among physicians of general medicine-related specialties [11].

The hematological features of CD include a variety of conditions—anemia, platelet alterations (thrombocytopenia/thrombocytosis), hemorrhagic or thrombotic events, IgA deficiency, hyposplenism, and the fearful lymphoma (Table 1) [12,13].

A high frequency of hematologic alterations (84%) has been reported in CD patients ever since decades ago [14]. Still, there is a high burden of missed CD cases and significant diagnostic delay in frequent clinical situations, such as chronic, unresponsive iron-deficiency anemia. Better recognition of the hematologic findings could be a window of opportunity to increase the diagnostic rate of CD, which is known to be severely underdiagnosed [15]. Although currently available guidelines from the American College of Gastroenterology (ACG), British Society of Gastroenterology (BSG), European Society for Pediatric Gastroenterology, Hepatology, and Nutrition (ESPGHAN), and European Society for the Study of Coeliac Disease (ESsCD) [16–19] approach some of these hematological features of CD, others are not very well reported.

Our aim was to perform a review of recent literature data regarding hematologic manifestations of CD and their management. For this purpose, we performed a literature search on two databases—PubMed and Embase—from 2010 onwards, using the MESH term "celiac disease" and several keywords referring to the associated hematological features: "hematology", "anemia", "thrombocytosis", "thrombocytopenia", "hemorrhage", "thrombosis", "coagulation", "IgA deficiency", "spleen", and "lymphoma". Articles identified from this search strategy were checked for access to abstract in English and then further evaluated for relevance to the topic. Clinically significant full-text articles were selected for inclusion in this review; also, references of selected articles were further checked for additional possible meaningful articles, which were not identified by the initial search.

In this review, updated knowledge regarding hematologic manifestations of CD is summarized in accordance with recent data published in the literature.

Table 1. Hematologic manifestations of celiac disease (CD).

Hematologic Feature	Frequency	Proposed Mechanism
Anemia	Common	Most frequently iron-deficiency, but may be also due to folate, B12 or copper deficiency
Thrombocytopenia	Rare	Autoimmunity
Thrombocytosis	Relatively common	Iron-deficiency, hyposplenism
Hemorrhagic events	Rare	Vitamin K deficiency
Thrombotic events	Rare	Hyperhomocystinemia, elevated levels of other procoagulants, protein C/S deficiency
Hyposplenism	Common	Autoimmunity
IgA deficiency	Relatively common	Associated conditions
Lymphoma	Rare	Refractory CD

2. Anemia

Anemia in CD patients is multifactorial in etiology; however, iron-deficiency anemia (IDA) is the most common reported [20]. Laboratory workup for IDA can reveal anemia, low mean corpuscular volume, low serum iron, low serum ferritin or anisocytosis (increased red blood cell distribution width) [21]. The main mechanism for IDA in CD is related to malabsorption, as the site of iron absorption—the proximal duodenum—is almost always involved [12]. Severity of iron malabsorption seems to be related to the extent of atrophy along the small bowel, as recent data on ultra-short CD (CD limited to the duodenal bulb) have reported lower proportion of ferritin deficiency in this group compared to extensive CD, both in children and adults [22,23]. Interestingly, anemia in CD is not only related to gluten-driven damage of the bowel mucosa, as it was also reported in patients with positive serology before development of atrophy [24]; this reinforces the need for CD testing in IDA patients and early recommendation of a gluten-free diet in these potential CD patients (the so called "celiac trait") with extraintestinal manifestations [25].

IDA is one of the most frequent extraintestinal presentations of CD and, according to current guidelines, is an indication for CD screening. According to a recent systematic review and meta-analysis, 3.2% of patients with IDA have biopsy-proven CD [26]. Conversely, up to half of newly diagnosed CD patients, both children and adults, have anemia [10,27–29]. In this setting, some authors have even proposed routine duodenal biopsies in IDA patients as a case finding strategy for CD, but this has not proven cost-effective [30–32]. As such, the first step in evaluating the suspicion of CD in IDA patients remains serological testing [33], as it is currently recommended in guidelines [34].

One of the characteristics of IDA in CD is refractoriness to oral iron supplements [35]. If symptomatic, correction of anemia can be done by intravenous iron; otherwise, it usually restores in parallel with the histological recovery of atrophic mucosa on gluten-free diet [36]. Lack of anemia correction on follow-up visits should prompt for search of other causes (colonoscopy, capsule endoscopy) and evaluation for refractory CD [37].

Sharing the same site of absorption as iron, folate deficiency can also occur in CD, leading to macrocytic (or normocytic when deficits are combined) anemia; additionally, we should take into account that normocytic anemia does not rule out IDA, as up to 40% of patients with IDA have normal mean corpuscular volume [38]. Studies have reported up to one fifth of patients having low folate levels [27].

Vitamin B12 deficiency was considered theoretically to be less common in CD, as its absorption takes place in the terminal ileum, which is infrequently involved. However, studies have reported significant proportions for B12 deficiency also [20,27].

Anemia of chronic disease, defined by anemia with high ferritin levels and inflammatory syndrome, has been also described in CD [39,40]. Associated aplastic anemia has also been reported in isolated cases [41–43].

3. Hemorrhagic and Thrombotic Events

Hemorrhagic events can be the presenting feature of CD, including cases of celiac crisis with profound malabsorption and coagulation deficits [44]. A recent review of the literature has found only case reports of hemorrhagic events, comprising otorhinolaryngology, digestive, urology, muscular and alveolar bleeding (the latter defining the Lane Hamilton syndrome) [45]. The mechanism behind hemorrhagic diathesis in CD is mainly represented by vitamin K deficiency, while some studies have also theorized mimicry between factor XIII and tissue transglutaminase [45,46]. Management of hemorrhage consists of intravenous vitamin K and GFD, along with specific measures according to bleeding site.

With respect to thrombotic events, they can also be the prime manifestation of CD. Most cases report on venous thrombosis (deep venous thrombosis, pulmonary embolism, cerebral venous thrombosis, intraabdominal thrombosis), while arterial events have been rarely described [12,47–50]. In addition to case reports, an increased risk of venous thromboembolism has been shown in large cohort studies [51]. Among the proposed mechanisms, hyperhomocystinemia, protein C/S deficiency, high titers of anti-phospholipid antibodies, and platelet abnormalities have been quoted [52,53].

Although rarer than anemia, hemorrhagic/thrombotic events as a manifestation of CD should be acknowledged accordingly, as they can be of significant clinical impact.

4. Lymphoma

CD patients are known to be at increased risk for developing malignancies [54]. Among them, lymphoma is the most fearful complication of CD, as it has a dismal prognosis. In a large population-based case-control study, the odds ratio for developing T-cell lymphoma after a prior diagnosis of CD was 35.8 (95% CI 27.1–47.4) [55]. Patients at risk for lymphoma are those with persistent villous atrophy, meaning those with refractory CD. The absolute risk of lymphoma, while increased, remains low—among 1000 patients with CD followed for 10 years, 7 out of 1000 will develop lymphoma, while the risk is 10/1000 in those with persistent villous atrophy and 4/1000 in healing (similar to that of general population) [56]. Management of lymphoma is multimodal oncologic treatment, but prognosis is often poor.

5. Hyposplenism and Susceptibility to Infections

Spleen dysfunction with hyposplenism has also been reported in CD patients. Its underlying mechanism seems to be related to antibody deposits in the spleen [57]. On a peripheral blood smear, one can find some characteristic changes of hyposplenism such as Howell–Jolly bodies, acanthocytes, and target cells [13].

Measuring spleen size is of interest in case of suspected/confirmed CD, as some small-sampled studies have linked splenic hypotrophy with CD and other have shown an association of small spleen volume with refractory CD [58–60].

Along with the changes in size, functional hyposplenism is of importance in CD patients, as it can lead to thrombocytosis and susceptibility to infections, especially encapsulated bacteria (*Streptococcus pneumoniae, Haemophilus influenzae, Neisseria meningitidis*) [13]. Immunization against these bacteria should be recommended in CD patients [61,62].

Susceptibility to infections is not only related to hyposplenism, as other factors may also contribute—malnutrition, vitamin D deficiency, altered mucosal permeability and gut microbiota. Increased rates of infections in CD patients have been reported for influenza, herpes zoster, pneumonia, tuberculosis, and Clostridium difficile [63–66]. However, the risk of infections requiring hospitalization does not seem to be influenced by mucosal healing [67].

6. IgA Deficiency

There is a strong association between CD and IgA deficiency, meaning that 2%–3% of CD patients have IgA deficiency and about 8% of individuals with IgA deficiency have CD [13]. Several clinical consequences arise: First, there is the susceptibility to develop other small-bowel diseases such as inflammatory bowel disease or parasite infections (Giardiasis for example, which can histologically mimic CD), then there is the issue regarding diagnosis of CD in these patients, as IgA-based serology can lead to false-negative results (for this reason testing for suspicion of CD includes total serum IgA dosing or both IgA and IgG-based serology), and last, there is a risk of serious transfusion reactions in patients with anti-IgA antibodies [68,69].

7. Conclusions

While classical presentations of CD with typical malabsorption syndrome are becoming exceptional, extraintestinal forms are now considered the predominant ones. Among the wide range of extraintestinal features, hematologic-related ones are quite frequent, and they can be the sole manifestation of the disease. IDA is the most frequent hematologic feature of CD, and screening for CD should not be missed in patients with unexplained and refractory to iron-supplementation IDA. Earlier markers of iron-deficiency (alteration in hematological indices of red blood cells) and also changes in platelet numbers should also prompt for testing in a suggestive clinical setting. Hemorrhagic or thrombotic events, otherwise unexplained, can also be the presenting feature of CD. Not least, IgA deficiency and evidence of small-bowel lymphoma should prompt for CD testing. A diagnosis of CD should be always kept in mind in front of a patient with unexplained hematologic abnormalities.

Author Contributions: Conceptualization—D.V.B.; Literature search—all co-authors; writing—original draft preparation, D.V.B.; writing—review and editing, A.P., F.I.R. and M.J.; supervision—A.P., F.I.R. and M.J.

Funding: This research received no external funding.

Conflicts of Interest: The authors declare no conflict of interest.

References

1. Gujral, N.; Freeman, H.J.; Thomson, A.B. Celiac disease: Prevalence, diagnosis, pathogenesis and treatment. *World J. Gastroenterol.* **2012**, *18*, 6036–6059. [CrossRef] [PubMed]
2. Singh, P.; Arora, A.; Strand, T.A.; Leffler, D.A.; Catassi, C.; Green, P.H.; Kelly, C.P.; Ahuja, V.; Makharia, G.K. Global prevalence of celiac disease: Systematic review and meta-analysis. *Clin. Gastroenterol. Hepatol.* **2018**, *16*, 823–836.e2. [CrossRef] [PubMed]
3. Leffler, D.A.; Green, P.H.; Fasano, A. Extraintestinal manifestations of coeliac disease. *Nat. Rev. Gastroenterol. Hepatol.* **2015**, *12*, 561–571. [CrossRef] [PubMed]
4. Reunala, T.; Salmi, T.T.; Hervonen, K.; Kaukinen, K.; Collin, P. Dermatitis Herpetiformis: A Common Extraintestinal Manifestation of Coeliac Disease. *Nutrients* **2018**, *10*, 602. [CrossRef] [PubMed]
5. Pinto-Sanchez, M.I.; Bercik, P.; Verdu, E.F.; Bai, J.C. Extraintestinal manifestations of celiac disease. *Dig. Dis.* **2015**, *33*, 147–154. [CrossRef] [PubMed]
6. Rodrigo, L.; Beteta-Gorriti, V.; Alvarez, N.; Gómez de Castro, C.; de Dios, A.; Palacios, L.; Santos-Juanes, J. Cutaneous and mucosal manifestations associated with celiac disease. *Nutrients* **2018**, *10*, 800. [CrossRef]
7. Dima, A.; Jurcut, C.; Jinga, M. Rheumatologic manifestations in celiac disease. *Rom. J. Intern. Med.* **2019**, *57*, 3–5.
8. Casella, G.; Bordo, B.M.; Shaclling, R.; Villanacci, V.; Salemme, M.; Di Bella, C.; Bassotti, G. Neurological disorders and celiac disease. *Minerva Gastroenterol. Dietol.* **2016**, *62*, 197–206.
9. Abenavoli, L.; Luigiano, C.; Larussa, T.; Milic, N.; De Lorenzo, A.; Stelitano, L.; Morace, C.; Consolo, P.; Miraglia, S.; Fagoonee, S.; et al. Liver steatosis in celiac disease: The open door. *Minerva Gastroenterol. Dietol.* **2013**, *59*, 89–95.
10. Catal, F.; Topal, E.; Ermistekin, H.; Acar, N.Y.; Sinanoğlu, M.S.; Karabiber, H.; Selimoğlu, M.A. The hematologic manifestations of pediatric celiac disease at the time of diagnosis and efficiency of gluten free diet. *Turk. J. Med. Sci.* **2015**, *45*, 663–667. [CrossRef]
11. Jinga, M.; Popp, A.; Balaban, D.V.; Dima, A.; Jurcut, C. Physicians' attitude and perception regarding celiac disease: A questionnaire-based study. *Turk. J. Gastroenterol.* **2018**, *29*, 419–426. [CrossRef] [PubMed]
12. Baydoun, A.; Maakaron, J.E.; Halawi, H.; Abou Rahal, J.; Taher, A.T. Hematological manifestations of celiac disease. *Scand. J. Gastroenterol.* **2012**, *47*, 1401–1411. [CrossRef] [PubMed]
13. Halfdanarson, T.R.; Litzow, M.R.; Murray, J.A. Hematologic manifestations of celiac disease. *Blood* **2007**, *109*, 412–421. [CrossRef] [PubMed]
14. Croese, J.; Harris, O.; Bain, B. Coeliac disease. Haematological features, and delay in diagnosis. *Med. J. Aust.* **1979**, *2*, 335–338. [PubMed]
15. Green, P.H. Where are all those patients with Celiac disease? *Am. J. Gastroenterol.* **2007**, *102*, 1461–1463. [CrossRef] [PubMed]
16. Rubio-Tapia, A.; Hill, I.D.; Kelly, C.P.; Calderwood, A.H.; Murray, J.A. American College of Gastroenterology. ACG clinical guidelines: Diagnosis and management of celiac disease. *Am. J. Gastroenterol.* **2013**, *108*, 656–676. [CrossRef] [PubMed]
17. Ludvigsson, J.F.; Bai, J.C.; Biagi, F.; Card, T.R.; Ciacci, C.; Ciclitira, P.J.; Green, H.R.; Hadjivassiliou, M.; Holdoway, A.; Van Hee, D.A.; et al. BSG Coeliac Disease Guidelines Development Group; British Society of Gastroenterology. Diagnosis and management of adult coeliac disease: Guidelines from the British Society of Gastroenterology. *Gut* **2014**, *63*, 1210–1228. [CrossRef] [PubMed]
18. Husby, S.; Koletzko, S.; Korponay-Szabó, I.R.; Mearin, M.L.; Phillips, A.; Shamir, R.; Troncone, R.; Giersiepen, K.; Branski, D.; Catassi, C.; et al. ESPGHAN Working Group on Coeliac Disease Diagnosis; ESPGHAN Gastroenterology Committee; European Society for Pediatric Gastroenterology, Hepatology, and Nutrition guidelines for the diagnosis of coeliac disease. *J. Pediatr. Gastroenterol. Nutr.* **2012**, *54*, 136–160. [CrossRef]
19. Al-Toma, A.; Volta, U.; Auricchio, R.; Castillejo, G.; Sanders, D.S.; Cellier, C.; Mulder, C.J.; Lundin, K.E.A. European Society for the Study of Coeliac Disease (ESsCD) guideline for coeliac disease and other gluten-related disorders. *UEG J.* **2019**, *7*, 583–613. [CrossRef]

20. Berry, N.; Basha, J.; Varma, N.; Varma, S.; Prasad, K.K.; Vaiphei, K.; Vaiphei, N.; Sinha, S.K.; Kochhar, R. Anemia in celiac disease is multifactorial in etiology: A prospective study from India. *JGH Open* **2018**, *2*, 196–200. [CrossRef]
21. Balaban, D.V.; Popp, A.; Beata, A.; Vasilescu, F.; Jinga, M. Diagnostic accuracy of red blood cell distribution width-to-lymphocyte ratio for celiac disease. *Rev. Romana Med. Lab.* **2018**, *26*, 45–50. [CrossRef]
22. Mooney, P.D.; Kurien, M.; Evans, K.E.; Rosario, E.; Cross, S.S.; Vergani, P.; Hadjivassiliou, M.; Murray, J.A.; Sanders, D.S. Clinical and immunologic features of ultra-short celiac disease. *Gastroenterology* **2016**, *150*, 1125–1134. [CrossRef] [PubMed]
23. Doyev, R.; Cohen, S.; Ben-Tov, A.; Weintraub, Y.; Amir, A.; GalaiHadar, T.; Moran-Lev, H.; Yerushalmy-Feler, A. Ultra-short celiac disease is a distinct and milder phenotype of the disease in children. *Dig. Dis. Sci.* **2019**, *64*, 167–172. [CrossRef] [PubMed]
24. Repo, M.; Lindfors, K.; Mäki, M.; Heini, H.; Kaija, L.; Marja-Leena, L.; Päivi, S.; Katri, S.; Kalle, K. Anemia and Iron Deficiency in Children with Potential Celiac Disease. *J. Pediatr. Gastroenterol. Nutr.* **2017**, *64*, 56–62. [CrossRef] [PubMed]
25. Popp, A.; Maki, M. Gluten-induced extra-intestinal manifestations in potential celiac disease-celiac trait. *Nutrients* **2019**, *11*, 320. [CrossRef] [PubMed]
26. Mahadev, S.; Laszkowska, M.; Sundstrom, J.; Björkholm, M.; Lebwohl, B.; Green, P.H.R.; Ludvigsson, J.F. Prevalence of celiac disease in patients with iron deficiency anemia—A systematic review and meta-analysis. *Gastroenterology* **2018**, *155*, 374–382. [CrossRef] [PubMed]
27. Wierdsma, N.J.; van Bokhorst-de van der Scheuren, M.A.; Berkenpas, M.; Mulder, C.J.J.; Van Bodegraven, A.A. Vitamin and mineral deficiencies are highly prevalent in newly diagnosed celiac disease patients. *Nutrients* **2013**, *5*, 3975–3992. [CrossRef]
28. Deora, V.; Aylward, N.; Sokoro, A.; El-Matary, W. Serum vitamins and minerals at diagnosis and follow-up in children with celiac disease. *J. Ped. Gastroenterol. Nutr.* **2017**, *65*, 185–189. [CrossRef]
29. Laurikka, P.; Nurminen, S.; Kivelä, L.; Kurppa, K. Extraintestinal manifestations of celiac disease: Early detection for better long-term outcomes. *Nutrients* **2018**, *10*, 1015. [CrossRef]
30. Herrod, P.J.J.; Lund, J.N. Random duodenal biopsy to exclude coeliac disease as a cause of anaemia is not cost-effective and should be replaced with universally performed pre-endoscopy serology in patients on a suspected cancer pathway. *Tech. Coloproctol.* **2018**, *22*, 121–124. [CrossRef]
31. Grisolano, S.W.; Oxentenko, A.S.; Murray, J.A.; Burgart, L.J.; Dierkhising, R.A.; Alexander, J.A. The usefulness of routine small bowel biopsies in evaluation of iron deficiency anaemia. *J. Clin. Gastroenterol.* **2004**, *38*, 756–760. [CrossRef] [PubMed]
32. Mandal, A.K.; Mehdi, I.; Munshi, S.K.; Lo, T.C. Value of routine duodenal biopsy in diagnosing coeliac disease in patients with iron deficiency anaemia. *Postgrad. Med. J.* **2004**, *80*, 475–477. [CrossRef] [PubMed]
33. Lau, M.S.; Mooney, P.; White, W.; Appleby, V.; Moreea, S.; Haythem, I.; Elias, J.E.; Bundhoo, K.; Corbett, G.D.; Wong, L.; et al. Pre-endoscopy point of care test (Simtomax- IgA/IgG-Deamidated Gliadin Peptide) for coeliac disease in iron deficiency anaemia: Diagnostic accuracy and a cost saving economic model. *BMC Gastroenterol.* **2016**, *16*, 115.
34. Goddard, A.F.; James, M.W.; McIntyre, A.S.; Scott, B.B. British Society of Gastroenterology. Guidelines for the management of iron deficiency anaemia. *Gut* **2011**, *60*, 1309–1316. [CrossRef] [PubMed]
35. Hershko, C.; Patz, J. Ironing out the mechanism of anemia in celiac disease. *Hematologica* **2008**, *93*, 1761–1765. [CrossRef] [PubMed]
36. Jericho, H.; Sansotta, N.; Guandalini, S. Extraintestinal Manifestations of Celiac Disease: Effectiveness of the Gluten-Free Diet. *J. Pediatr. Gastroenterol. Nutr.* **2017**, *65*, 75–79. [CrossRef]
37. Hopper, A.D.; Leeds, J.S.; Hurlstone, D.P.; Hadjivassiliou, M.; Drew, K.; Sanders, D.S. Are lower gastrointestinal investigations necessary in patients with coeliac disease? *Eur. J. Gastroenterol. Hepatol.* **2005**, *17*, 617–621. [CrossRef]
38. Johnson-Wimbley, T.D.; Graham, D.Y. Diagnosis and management of iron deficiency anemia in the 21st century. *Adv. Gastroenterol.* **2011**, *4*, 177–184. [CrossRef]
39. Harper, J.W.; Holleran, S.F.; Ramakrishnan, R.; Bhagat, G.; Green, P.H. Anemia in celiac disease is multifactorial in etiology. *Am. J. Hematol.* **2007**, *82*, 996–1000. [CrossRef]

40. Bergamaschi, G.; Markopoulos, K.; Albertini, R.; Sabatino, A.D.; Biag, F.; Ciccocioppo, R.; Arbustini, E.; Corazza, G.R. Anemia of chronic disease and defective erythropoetin production in patients with celiac disease. *Hematologica* **2008**, *93*, 1785–1791. [CrossRef]
41. Badyal, R.K.; Sachdeva, M.U.; Varma, N.; Thapa, B.R. A rare association of celiac disease and aplastic anemia: Case report of a child a review of the literature. *Pediatr. Dev. Pathol.* **2014**, *17*, 470–473. [CrossRef] [PubMed]
42. Basu, A.; Ray, Y.; Bowmik, P.; Rahman, M.; Dikshit, N.; Goswami, R.P. Rare association of coeliac disease with aplastic anemia. report of a case from India. *Indian J. Hematol. Blood Transfus.* **2014**, *30*, 208–211. [CrossRef] [PubMed]
43. Chatterjee, S.; Dey, P.K.; Roy, P.; Sinha, M.K. Celiac disease with pure red cell aplasia: An unusual hematologic association in pediatric age group. *Indian J. Hematol. Blood Transfus.* **2014**, *30*, 383–385. [CrossRef] [PubMed]
44. Balaban, D.V.; Dima, A.; Jurcut, C.; Popp, A.; Jinga, M. Celiac crisis, a rare occurrence in adult celiac disease: A systematic review. *World J. Clin. Cases* **2019**, *7*, 311–319. [CrossRef] [PubMed]
45. Dima, A.; Jurcut, C.; Manolache, A.; Balaban, D.V.; Popp, A.; Jinga, M. Hemorrhagic Events in Adult Celiac Disease Patients. Case Report and Review of the Literature. *J. Gastrointestin. Liver Dis.* **2018**, *27*, 93–99. [PubMed]
46. Sjöber, K.; Eriksson, S.; Tenngart, B.; Roth, E.B.; Leffler, H.; Stenberg, P. Factor XIII and tissue transglutaminase antibodies in coeliac and inflammatory bowel disease. *Autoimmunity* **2002**, *35*, 357–364. [CrossRef] [PubMed]
47. Dumic, I.; Martin, S.; Salfiti, N.; Watson, R.; Alempijevic, T. Deep Venous Thrombosis and Bilateral Pulmonary Embolism Revealing Silent Celiac Disease: Case Report and Review of the Literature. *Case Rep. Gastrointest. Med.* **2017**, *2017*, 5236918. [CrossRef] [PubMed]
48. Ciaccio, E.J.; Lewis, S.K.; Biviano, A.; Iyer, V.; Garan, H.; Green, P.H. Cardiovascular involvement in celiac disease. *World J. Cardiol.* **2017**, *9*, 652–666. [CrossRef] [PubMed]
49. Beyrouti, R.; Mansour, M.; Kacem, A.; Derbali, H.; Mrissa, R. Recurrent cerebral venous thrombosis revealing celiac disease: An exceptional case report. *Acta Neurol. Belg.* **2017**, *117*, 341–343. [CrossRef]
50. Meena, D.S.; Sonwal, V.S.; Bohra, G.K. Celiac disease with Budd-Chiari syndrome: A rare association. *SAGE Open Med. Case Rep.* **2019**, *7*, 1–3. [CrossRef]
51. Ludvigsson, J.F.; Welander, A.; Lassila, R.; Ekbom, A.; Montgomery, S.M. Risk of thromboembolism in 14,000 individuals with coeliac disease. *Br. J. Haematol.* **2007**, *139*, 121–127. [CrossRef] [PubMed]
52. Lerner, A.; Blank, M. Hypercoagulability in celiac disease—An update. *Autoimmun. Rev.* **2014**, *13*, 1138–1141. [CrossRef] [PubMed]
53. Laine, O.; Pitkanen, K.; Lindfors, K.; Huhtala, H.; Niemela, O.; Collin, P.; Kurppa, K.; Kaukinen, K. Elevated serum antiphospholipid antibodies in adults with celiac disease. *Dig. Liver Dis.* **2018**, *50*, 457–461. [CrossRef] [PubMed]
54. Han, Y.; Chen, W.; Li, P.; Ye, J. Association between coeliac disease and risk of any malignancy and gastrointestinal malignancy: A meta-analysis. *Medicine (Baltimore)* **2015**, *94*, e1612. [CrossRef] [PubMed]
55. Van Gils, T.; Nijeboer, P.; Overbeek, L.I.; Castelijn, D.A.; Bouma, G.; Mulder, C.J.; van Leeuwen, F.E.; de Jong, D. Risk of lymphomas and gastrointestinal carcinomas after a diagnosis of celiac disease based on a nationwide population-based case-control. study. *United Eur. Gastroenterol. J.* **2017**, *5* (Suppl. 1), A50. [CrossRef]
56. Lebwohl, B.; Granath, F.; Ekbom, A.; Smedby, K.E.; Murray, J.A.; Neugut, A.I.; Green, P.H.R.; Ludvigsson, J.F. Mucosal healing and risk for lymphoproliferative malignancy in celiac disease: A population-based cohort study. *Ann. Intern. Med.* **2013**, *159*, 169–175. [CrossRef] [PubMed]
57. Korponay-Szabó, I.R.; Halttunen, T.; Szalai, Z.; Laurila, K.; Király, R.; Kovács, J.B.; Fésüs, L.; Mäki, M. In vivo targeting of intestinal and extraintestinal transglutaminase 2 by coeliac autoantibodies. *Gut* **2004**, *53*, 641–648. [CrossRef] [PubMed]
58. Van Gils, T.; Nijeboer, P.; van Waesberghe, J.H.T.; Coupé, V.M.; Janssen, K.; Zegers, J.A.; Nurmohamed, S.A.; Kraal, G.; Jiskoot, S.C.; Bouma, G. Splenic volume differentiates complicated and non-complicated celiac disease. *UEG J.* **2017**, *5*, 374–379. [CrossRef] [PubMed]
59. Di Sabatino, A.; Brunetti, L.; Carnevale Maffè, G.; Giuffrida, P.; Corazza, G.R. Is it worth investigating splenic function in patients with celiac disease. *World J. Gastroenterol.* **2013**, *19*, 2313–2318. [CrossRef]
60. Balaban, D.V.; Popp, A.; Lungu, A.M.; Costache, R.S.; Anca, I.A.; Jinga, M. Ratio of spleen diameter to red blood cell distribution width: A novel indicator for celiac disease. Medicine (Baltimore). *Medicine* **2015**, *94*, e726. [CrossRef]

61. Canova, C.; Ludvigsson, J.; Baldo, V.; Amidei, C.B.; Zanier, A.; Zingone, F. Risk of bacterial pneumonia and pneymococcal infection in youths with celiac disease-A population-based study. *Dig. Liver Dis.* **2019**. [CrossRef] [PubMed]
62. Simons, M.; Scott-Sheldon, L.A.J.; Risech-Neyman, Y.; Moss, S.F.; Ludvigsson, J.F.; Green, P.H.R. Celiac disease and increased risk of pneumococcal infection: A systematic review and meta-analysis. *Am. J. Med.* **2018**, *131*, 83–89. [CrossRef] [PubMed]
63. Ludvigsson, J.; Choung, R.S.; Marietta, E.V.; Murray, J.A.; Emilsson, E. Increased risk of herpes zoster in patients with coeliac disease-nationwide cohort study. *Scand. J. Public Health* **2018**, *46*, 859–866. [CrossRef] [PubMed]
64. Lebwohl, B.; Nobel, Y.R.; Green, P.H.R.; Blaser, M.J.; Ludvigsson, J.F. Risk of Clostridium difficile Infection in Patients with Celiac Disease: A Population-Based Study. *Am. J. Gastroenterol.* **2017**, *112*, 1878–1884. [CrossRef] [PubMed]
65. Walters, J.R.; Bamford, K.B.; Ghosh, S. Coeliac disease and the risk of infections. *Gut* **2008**, *57*, 1034–1035. [CrossRef] [PubMed]
66. Ludvigsson, J.F.; Sanders, D.S.; Maeurer, M.; Jonsson, J.; Grunewald, J.; Wahlstrom, J. Risk of tuberculosis in a large sample of patients with celiac disease-a nationwide cohort study. *Aliment. Pharm.* **2011**, *33*, 689–696. [CrossRef] [PubMed]
67. Emilsson, L.; Lebwohl, B.; Green, P.H.; Murray, J.A.; Mårild, K.; Ludvigsson, J.F. Mucosal healing and the risk of serious infections in patients with celiac disease. *United Eur. Gastroenterol. J.* **2018**, *6*, 55–62. [CrossRef]
68. Wang, N.; Truedsson, L.; Elvin, K.; Andersson, B.A.; Rönnelid, J.; Mincheva-Nilsson, L.; Lindkvist, A.; Ludvigsson, J.F.; Hammarström, L.; Dahle, C. Serological assessment for celiac disease in IgA deficient adults. *PLoS ONE* **2014**, *9*, e93180. [CrossRef]
69. Vassallo, R.R. Review: IgA anaphylactic transfusion reactions, part I: Laboratory diagnosis, incidence, and supply of IgA-deficient products. *Immunohematology* **2004**, *20*, 226–233.

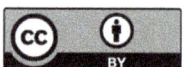

© 2019 by the authors. Licensee MDPI, Basel, Switzerland. This article is an open access article distributed under the terms and conditions of the Creative Commons Attribution (CC BY) license (http://creativecommons.org/licenses/by/4.0/).

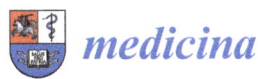

Review

Micronutrients Dietary Supplementation Advices for Celiac Patients on Long-Term Gluten-Free Diet with Good Compliance: A Review

Mariangela Rondanelli [1,2], Milena A. Faliva [3], Clara Gasparri [3], Gabriella Peroni [3], Maurizio Naso [3], Giulia Picciotto [3], Antonella Riva [4], Mara Nichetti [3], Vittoria Infantino [5], Tariq A. Alalwan [6] and Simone Perna [6,*]

1. IRCCS Mondino Foundation, 27100 Pavia, Italy
2. Department of Public Health, Experimental and Forensic Medicine, University of Pavia, 27100 Pavia, Italy
3. Endocrinology and Nutrition Unit, Azienda di Servizi alla Persona "Istituto Santa Margherita", University of Pavia, 27100 Pavia, Italy
4. Research and Development Unit, Indena, 20139 Milan, Italy
5. University of Bari, Department of Biomedical Science and Human Oncology, 70121 Bari, Italy
6. Department of Biology, College of Science, University of Bahrain, Sakhir Campus P. O. Box 32038, Bahrain
* Correspondence: sperna@uob.edu.bh; Tel.: +973 39 37 99 46

Received: 24 April 2019; Accepted: 27 June 2019; Published: 3 July 2019

Abstract: *Background and objective*: Often micronutrient deficiencies cannot be detected when patient is already following a long-term gluten-free diet with good compliance (LTGFDWGC). The aim of this narrative review is to evaluate the most recent literature that considers blood micronutrient deficiencies in LTGFDWGC subjects, in order to prepare dietary supplementation advice (DSA). *Materials and methods*: A research strategy was planned on PubMed by defining the following keywords: celiac disease, vitamin B12, iron, folic acid, and vitamin D. *Results*: This review included 73 studies. The few studies on micronutrient circulating levels in long-term gluten-free diet (LTGFD) patients over 2 years with good compliance demonstrated that deficiency was detected in up to: 30% of subjects for vitamin B12 (DSA: 1000 mcg/day until level is normal, then 500 mcg), 40% for iron (325 mg/day), 20% for folic acid (1 mg/day for 3 months, followed by 400–800 mcg/day), 25% for vitamin D (1000 UI/day or more-based serum level or 50,000 UI/week if level is <20 ng/mL), 40% for zinc (25–40 mg/day), 3.6% of children for calcium (1000–1500 mg/day), 20% for magnesium (200–300 mg/day); no data is available in adults for magnesium. *Conclusions*: If integration with diet is not enough, starting with supplements may be the correct way, after evaluating the initial blood level to determine the right dosage of supplementation.

Keywords: celiac disease; vitamin B12; iron; folic acid; vitamin D; long-term GFD therapy (LTGFD); LTGFD with good compliance (LTGFDWGC)

1. Introduction

Celiac disease (CD) is an immune-mediated systemic disorder triggered by the ingestion of gluten and prolamines in genetically predisposed individuals. It is characterized by inflammation of the small bowel mucosa—the immune reaction—which occurs after ingestion of gluten that leads to intestinal villous atrophy, crypt hyperplasia, and increased number of intraepithelial lymphocytes [1]. CD is a multifactorial disease and its pathogenesis involves both genetic and environmental factors [2]. Genetic composition for the development of the disease is evident. In fact, more than 90% of celiac patients are human leukocyte antigen (HLA)-DQ2 haplotype positive and almost all of the rest carry HLA-DQ8. These genes are necessary but not sufficient for CD development [3,4]. The predisposing

DQ2 and DQ8 heterodimers are composed of the association of α and β chains. A recent meta-analysis showed that the HLA genotypes coding for DQ2 or DQ8 heterodimers, but also those including only the alleles of the respective β chains (regardless of the concomitant presence of DQ2 or DQ8 α chains) have an increased risk of developing pediatric CD [5]. Recently, another meta-analysis evaluated the predictive values of HLA-DQB1*02 allele, suggesting the major relevance of this specific allele, rather than the expression of the full DQ2 and/or DQ8 heterodimers, in raising the risk to develop pediatric CD [6]. In addition, a risk gradient according to single or double copy of HLA-DQB1*02 has been revealed [6]. Gluten ingestion represents the major environmental factor, contributing to the development of the pathology, but there are several other conditions involved in the etiology of CD, including viral infections, gut microbiota, breastfeeding, early life feeding practice, and smoking [3,4].

CD can occur at any stage of life and with a great variety of signs and symptoms. In fact, it is considered a multisystem immunological disorder rather than a disease restricted only to the gastrointestinal tract. Consequently, it is important to make diagnosis not only in individuals with classic gastrointestinal symptoms, but also in subjects who have a more nuanced or extra-intestinal clinical features, since the consequences can be important in both cases [2]. To date, nutritional therapy has been the only effective treatment for patients with CD that demands a strict compliance with a gluten-free diet (GFD). Non-adherence to the GFD increases the risk of morbidity and mortality, as a result of associated conditions, which include infertility, skeletal disorders and malignancy. Once diagnosed, patients should be tested for micronutrient deficiencies, including iron, folic acid, vitamin B12, and vitamin D [7].

The 2013 American College of Gastroenterology guidelines reported that micronutrient deficiencies (in particular iron, folic acid, vitamins B6 and B12, vitamin D, copper, and zinc) are frequent in celiac patients at the time of celiac diagnosis. Therefore, patients with newly diagnosed celiac disease, micronutrient deficiencies should be found and integrated. These tests should include iron, folic acid, vitamin D, vitamin B12 and more [7].

Following the United Kingdom 2015 National Institute for Health and Care Excellence guidelines, it was reported that some patients with celiac disease may need additional nutritional supplements, mainly in the early stages after diagnosis, suggesting, however, that this should be identified through an appropriate ongoing monitoring and that integration should begin after a full evaluation [8].

These two guidelines are derived from, and in agreement with, the more recent reviews demonstrating that in celiac patients, at time of diagnosis, nutritional deficiencies are often found in vitamins and minerals, such as folic acid, vitamin B12, vitamin D, calcium, magnesium and zinc.

However, at the same time, in subjects undergoing GFD for a long time with good compliance, it has been described that micronutrient deficiencies may persist due to an inadequate full reintegration of the mucous membrane [9]. Some patients with long-term treated CD may still have abnormal small bowel mucosa and persistent villous atrophy on follow-up, with or without ongoing or recurrent symptoms, despite an apparently GFD [4,10]. According to Lanzini et al., the complete recovery of duodenal mucosa with histological normalization, after a median 16 months GFD in patients diagnosed at an adult age occurs only in 8% of cases [11]. The majority of adult patients achieving remission with intraepithelial lymphocytosis (65%) and a substantial proportion showing no-change (26%) or deterioration (1%) of duodenal histology [11]. This condition seems to be more common in adults older than an age of 50 years [12], but occurs even in 19% of children who underwent follow-up biopsy at least 1 year after starting the GFD [13]. When other possible causes of villous atrophy are excluded, refractory celiac disease is diagnosed [4]. Even in the absence of symptoms this condition is not positive, because it may predispose to severe complications, such as osteoporosis and malignancy [14].

Moreover, gluten-free products are usually low in some micronutrients, such as magnesium and folic acid, and gluten-free cereals found in nature have a lower magnesium content compared with gluten-containing ones [9].

This topic is highly debated in the literature. In fact, there is a widespread agreement on the importance of supplementation at the time of diagnosis, but there is still no consensus for when and what additional nutrients are needed in subjects on long-term GFD (LTGFD).

Given this background, the aim of this narrative review is to evaluate the literature that considers blood nutritional deficiencies in celiac subjects on LTGFD therapy with good compliance (LTGFDWGC) in order to prepare dietary supplementation advice for these patients.

2. Materials and Methods

The present narrative review was performed following the steps by Egger et al. [15] as follows:

1. Configuration of a working group: three operators skilled in clinical nutrition (one acting as a methodological operator and two participating as clinical operators).
2. Formulation of the revision question on the basis of considerations made in the abstract: "the state of the art on nutritional deficiencies in celiac subjects on LTGFD therapy with good compliance; "good compliance" was defined as those patients who had been apparently carefully compliant with the GFD for a at least one year based on dietary history, and this was supported by the absence of coeliac antibodies (if present at diagnosis), or having a healed duodenal biopsy if previous coeliac serology was unavailable".
3. Identification of relevant studies: a research strategy was planned on PubMed (Public MedIine run by the National Center of Biotechnology Information (NCBI) of the National Library of Medicine of Bathesda (USA)) as follows: (a) Definition of the keywords (celiac disease; vitamin B12; iron; folic acid; vitamin D; calcium; zinc; magnesium; LTGFD therapy; LTGFDWGC), allowing the definition of the interest field of the documents to be searched, grouped in quotation marks (" ... ") and used separately or in combination; (b) use of: the Boolean (a data type with only two possible values: true or false) AND operator, that allows the establishments of logical relations among concepts; (c) Research modalities: advanced search; (d) Limits: time limits: papers published in the last 20 years; humans; adults; languages: English; (e) Manual search performed by the senior researchers experienced in clinical nutrition through the revision of reviews and individual articles on management of inflammation and oxidative stress by dietary approach in celiac patients published in journals qualified in the Index Medicus.
4. Analysis and presentation of the outcomes: we create paragraphs about different micronutrients, and the data extrapolated from the "revised studies" were collocated in tables; in particular, for each study we specified the author and year of publication and study characteristics.
5. The analysis was carried out in the form of a narrative review of the reports. At the beginning of each section, the keywords considered and the type of studies chosen are reported. We evaluated, as is suitable for the narrative review, studies of any design which considered the nutritional deficiencies in celiac adult subjects on LTGFD therapy with good compliance.

3. Results

This review included 73 eligible studies and the dedicated flowchart is shown in Figure 1.

Table 1 shows the reviews made on nutrient deficiencies in celiac patients at time of diagnosis and after LTGFDWGC.

Table S1 shows the studies concerning circulating levels and supplementation of micronutrients in celiac patients after LTGFDWGC.

The literature shows that nutritional deficiencies, considered by evaluating the blood values of these micronutrients, in celiac subjects on LTGFD with good compliance, relate to vitamin B12, folic acid, vitamin D, calcium, iron, magnesium, zinc, selenium, thiamine, riboflavin, niacin and vitamin K (Table 1).

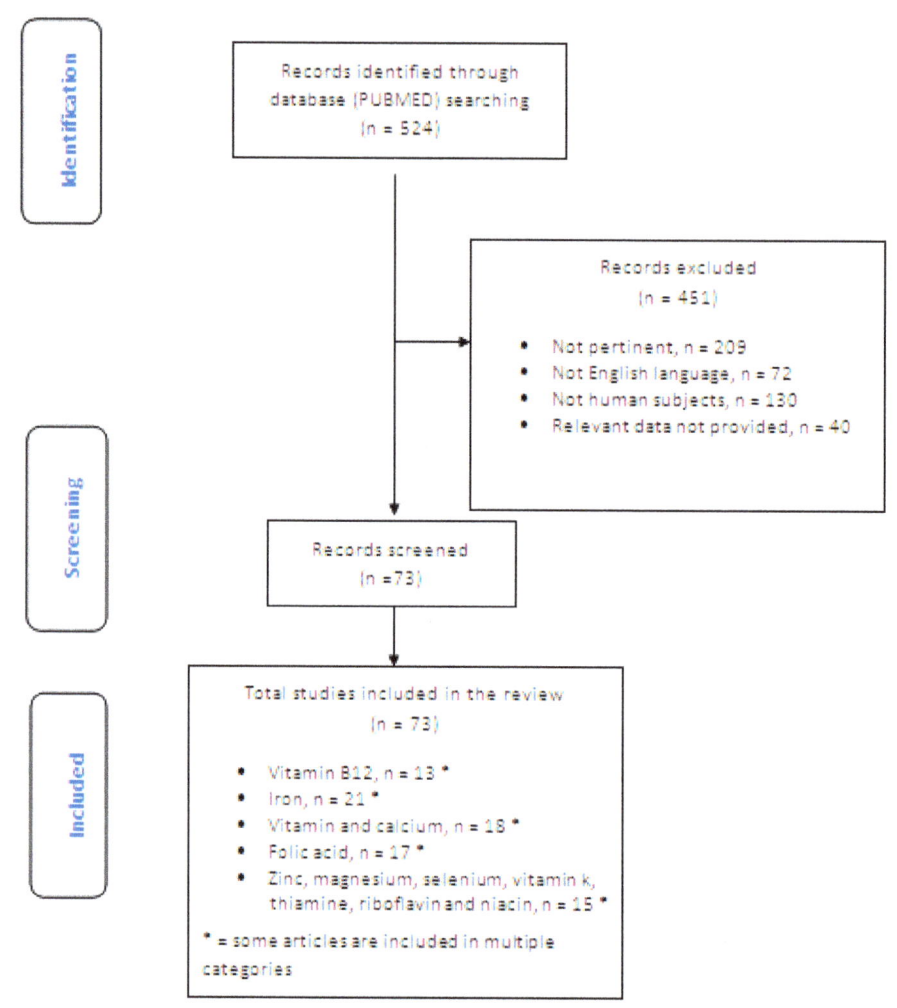

Figure 1. Flowchart of the study.

Table 1. Reviews on nutrient deficiencies in celiac patients at time of diagnosis and after GFD.

Authors	Type of Study	Country and Year	Results
[2]	Review	Italy, 2010	Common nutrient deficiencies in celiac subjects at diagnosis are: iron, calcium, magnesium, vitamin D, zinc, folate, niacin, vitamin B12, riboflavin, calorie/protein, and fiber. Deficiencies in folate, niacin, and vitamin B12 may occur after LTGFD.
[9]	Review	Italy, 2016	Low levels of fibers, folate, vitamin B12, vitamin D, calcium, iron, zinc and magnesium are common at diagnosis stage. In some subsets of treated celiac disease (CD) patients they can persist.

Table 1. *Cont.*

Authors	Type of Study	Country and Year	Results
[16]	Review	USA, 2005	Deficiencies in fiber, iron, calcium, vitamin D, magnesium, zinc, folate, niacin, vitamin B12, and riboflavin can occur at time of diagnosis. Deficiencies in fiber, iron, calcium, vitamin D, and magnesium can persist after following a GFD. Diet and gluten-free products are often low in B vitamins, calcium, vitamin D, iron, zinc, magnesium, and fiber.
[17]	Review	Italy, 2013	Reduced levels of iron, folate, vitamin B12, and vitamin D are common at the time of diagnosis. After GFD low levels of folate, vitamin B12 and vitamin D can persist.
[18]	Review	Italy, 2013	Common deficiencies at diagnosis include: fiber, iron, calcium, vitamin D, magnesium, zinc, folate, niacin, and vitamin B12. Deficiencies of fiber, iron, calcium, vitamin D, magnesium, zinc, folate, niacin, vitamin B12 may persist after following a GFD. Deficiencies of fiber, folate, niacin, vitamin B12, and riboflavin may persist after LTGFD.

3.1. Vitamin B12

This research was carried out based on the keywords "vitamin B12" AND "supplementation" AND "long-term GFD with good compliance" AND "celiac patient" OR "celiac disease". Of the 13 studies that were taken into account, 6 were review-type papers, 3 were prospective studies, 2 were observational studies and 2 were randomized controlled trials.

The absorption of dietary vitamin B12 occurs mainly in the terminal ileum through an active, specific and saturable transport mechanism. Vitamin B12 is released from food proteins after exposure to gastric acid. Vitamin B12 links to a salivary and gastric R protein; then pancreatic proteases destroy the R protein in the duodenum, releasing cobalamin which creates a complex with intrinsic factor (IF) that is secreted by the parietal cells in the stomach. The complex B12-FI migrates up to the terminal ileum aided by intestinal peristalsis, and binds itself through its proteic fraction to a specific cellular receptor. The complex dissociates and cobalamin enters the enterocytes of the small intestine. When the vitamin is administered orally in high doses, a small proportion along the entire intestine is absorbed through a passive diffusion mechanism.

Absorption site remains relatively preserved in patients with CD, so deficiency of vitamin B12 should be unusual. Nevertheless, numerous studies have shown that circulating levels of this vitamin are inadequate in about 5–40% of patients with CD at diagnosis [19–22] and in about 2.9-41% of patients following a GFD [20,21].

A real link exists between CD and vitamin B12 deficiency, but it has not been established. Some studies have shown that GFD and, where required, supplementation with vitamin B12 is effective in resolving neurological complications associated with deficiency of this vitamin. It has been shown that concentration of vitamin B12 tends to normalize in patients with a LTGFD [17,23].

However, there is evidence that supplementation may also be useful in subjects undergoing GFD. Hallert et al. [24] conducted a double-blind study to evaluate the effects of supplementation with B vitamins in adult CD patients for a long time, which involved daily administration of 0.8 mg of folic acid, 0.5 mg of cyanocobalamin, and 3 mg of pyridoxine for a period of 6 months. In these patients, there was improvement of psychiatric symptoms, and a significant return to normal vitamin B12 values with reduction of homocysteine values, which is often elevated in patients with vitamin B12 deficiency. Indeed, the catabolism of homocysteine requires vitamin B12 and folate. Consequently, hyperhomocysteinemia may reflect a deficit of both nutrients [25]. Great attention to the levels of homocysteine is needed in patients with CD. Celiac patients appear to have an increased risk of venous thromboembolism and vascular disorders [26] and high levels of homocysteine is a risk factor for these chronic diseases [27]. Supplementation of vitamin B12 and folate tends to decrease homocysteine values [24], so it could represent a prevention behavior.

In some patients, it is therefore necessary to integrate this element, even when following a strict GFD. In such cases, administration of vitamin B12 can be given via the oral or intramuscular routes.

In a study carried out by Bolaman et al. on general populations with megaloblastic anemia due to deficiency of cobalamin, oral supplementation was as effective as intramuscular treatment. Oral administration seems to be less costly and more tolerable than intramuscular delivery [28]. Furthermore, a review carried out by Vidal-Alaball et al. on general populations showed that in patients with a deficiency of vitamin B12, oral administration of 2000 mcg/day or 1000 mcg/day, followed by 1000 mcg/week and then 1000 mcg/month, can be as effective as intramuscular administration in showing improvement in hematological and neurological levels [29].

In patients with CD, supplementation is recommended for those in which there remains a blood deficiency despite GFD. Hallert et al. have shown how the oral administration of 500 mcg of cyanocobalamin in subjects undergoing GFD is effective in restoring the homocysteine value (which is an indirect measurement of vitamin B12 and folate). It suggests that the absorption after oral administration, especially in subjects undergoing GFD, is effective [24]. Furthermore, Theethira et al. suggested measuring vitamin B12 levels at diagnosis and then every 1–2 years for symptoms, and to treat with 1000 mcg orally until levels normalize, and then considering daily gluten-free multi vitamin/mineral supplementation [30].

In conclusion, considering the site of absorption (terminal ileum) of vitamin B12, which remains relatively preserved in patients with CD, deficiency of this vitamin should be infrequent; however, circulating levels of this vitamin could remain inadequate up to 41% in LTGGFDWGC patients. Given this background, in addition to its pivotal role in preventing hyperomocysteinemia, an annual routine follow-up of blood vitamin B12 level is mandatory in subjects undergoing LTGFD. Regarding dose and route of administration, the literature showed that in celiac patients with vitamin B12 deficiency, oral administration of 1000 mcg of vitamin B12 until levels normalized, followed by daily gluten-free multi-vitamin/mineral supplementation with 500 mcg of vitamin B12 is effective [30].

3.2. Iron

This research was carried out based on the keywords "iron" AND "supplementation" AND "long-term GFD with good compliance" AND "celiac patient" OR "celiac disease". Of the 21 studies that were taken into consideration, 8 were prospective studies, 5 were reviews, 3 were observational case studies, 2 were case control studies, 1 was a randomized controlled trial, 1 was a report and 1 was a guidelines.

Iron deficiency often occurs in celiac patients, and it is followed in many cases by iron deficiency anemia. Studies have shown that the prevalence of this event in patients with newly diagnosed CD seems to be between 10–80%. The prevalence of deficiency after 6 months of GFD is about 70%, after 1 year, it is about 50%, and after 2 years, it is about 40% [17,19,31–37].

Iron is an essential trace element, being part of the heme structure, the non-protein component of numerous iron proteins (such as hemoglobin, myoglobin and cytochromes). Its excretion cannot be controlled, so the amount of iron in the body depends mainly on its absorption, which takes place in the duodenum and proximal jejunum.

Iron deficiency anemia in CD patients mainly arises from malabsorption, although the possibility of intestinal bleeding cannot be excluded and must be considered [38,39].

In the general population, initial treatment of iron deficiency should be continued until hemoglobin and iron stores are normalized. This goal is usually obtained with oral iron administration. Although it is occasionally recommended to take iron supplements before breakfast in order to increase the absorption, this significantly reduces the tolerance. For this reason, it seems reasonable to suggest the administration with food. All ferrous salts, including ferrous fumarate, ferrous lactate, ferrous succinate, ferrous glutamate, and ferrous sulphate, share similar bioavailability. Preparations of iron glycinate represent a valid therapeutic alternative, since they have a good bioavailability and a lower frequency of side effects, such as constipation [40–42].

Treatment with oral iron is, in the general population, slow in reaching its goal, and good compliance is required to be successful. In addition to this, anemia is often severe, and a quick response is necessary. Sometimes the tolerance is poor, and in these situations the use of parenteral iron is fully justified. The efficacy and safety of parenteral iron sucrose use have been demonstrated in several clinical studies and have been confirmed by extensive clinical practice [43]. To supply the quantities required, several doses are needed. Other intravenous drugs such as ferric carboxymaltose have been introduced [44] and would require fewer infusions to provide the required dose. Ferric carboxymaltose is a robust and stable non-dextran intravenous iron formulation with the advantage of having a very low immunogenic potential, and therefore is not predisposed to anaphylactic reactions. Its properties permit the administration of large doses (15 mg/kg; maximum of 1000 mg/infusion) in a single and rapid session (15-min infusion) [45].

Therapy on the general population should start with a low dose and the intake should be constant until the iron deposits are not restored [40]. It is fundamental that treatment of an underlying cause should prevent further iron loss, but all patients should have iron supplementation, both to correct anemia and to replenish body stores. This is achieved most simply and cheaply with oral ferrous sulphate 200 mg twice daily. Lower doses may be as effective and better tolerated, and should be considered in patients not tolerating traditional doses. Other iron compounds (e.g., ferrous fumarate, ferrous gluconate) or formulations (iron suspensions) may also be tolerated better than ferrous sulphate. Oral iron should be continued for 3 months after the iron deficiency has been corrected so that stores are replenished [46].

Regarding celiac patients, in subjects in which iron supplementation is needed, it should be started orally. In the decision on when to start, some authors suggest undertaking supplementation in the moment in which the intestinal lesions are healed [40], while other studies suggest taking the supplement immediately at the time of diagnosis, without waiting for the healing of the mucosa [47]. In most of these patients, GFD is enough to solve the framework of anemia [48], although it may take a long time. In other cases it is necessary to help the patient with supplementation [36]. A study carried out on 25 pediatric patients with CD and iron deficiency showed good efficacy of oral administration of iron, (investigated with ferrous bisglycinate chelate 0.5 mg per kg body weight, reaching a maximum of 28 mg) both in patients with GFD and in those newly diagnosed [47]. A study carried out on celiac pediatric patients showed that the therapeutic dose in pediatric patients with an iron deficiency is 3 mg of elemental iron per kg body weight per day. The prophylactic dose in pediatric patients is 2 mg of elemental iron per kg body weight per day reaching a maximum dosage of 30 mg per day [36].

Since gluten-free products are characterized by a low iron content [49], the intake of foods rich in this mineral, such as meat, should be recommended to patients initiating a GFD.

Theethira et al. suggested measuring serum iron and ferritin at diagnosis, repeating every 3–6 months until ferritin was normal, and then every 1–2 years for symptoms. Moreover, they suggested iron supplements (325 mg), 1–3 tablets based on initial ferritin level until iron stores are restored, and consideration of intravenous (IV) iron for severe symptomatic iron deficiency anemia or intolerance of oral iron.

In conclusion, it seems that when long GFD, including food tips to consume adequate dietary iron, is not enough to restore iron levels (40% of LTGFDWGC subjects are iron-deficient), the right approach could be to start with oral administration of iron.

Based on this background, a semi-annual steady and routine follow-up of blood iron and ferritin levels is mandatory in subjects undergoing LTGFD [30].

3.3. Folic Acid

This research was carried out based on the keywords "folic acid" AND "supplementation" AND "long-term GFD with good compliance" AND "celiac patient" OR "celiac disease". A total of 17 studies were taken into consideration. Among these studies, 7 were prospective studies, 5 were review studies, 2 were observational case studies, 2 were randomized controlled trials, and 1 was a report.

The term "folate" describes the vitamer group B, based on the main structure of folic acid, which shares the same vitamin activity. This group of vitamins is essential for the synthesis and repairing of DNA, and they also act as cofactors for the enzymes involved in several biological reactions. Folate occurs naturally in some foods, and its synthetic form, folic acid, is added to many food products to increase the dietary intake. An example of supplementation is the addition of folic acid to wheat flour, which has been introduced in 52 countries worldwide since 2007 [50].

Folate deficiency was detected in about 10–85% of adult patients with CD at diagnosis, and in about 0-20% of patients following a GFD [17,20,22,51–54]. Usually the folate deficiency in CD occurs in patients with lesions in the ileum [48,55,56].

Tighe et al. compared in the general population the effectiveness of 0.2 mg folic acid per day with that of 0.4 and 0.8 mg/day in lowering homocysteine concentrations over a 6-month period. It has been seen that folic acid significantly reduces the risk of stroke overall by 18%, but to a greater extent by up to 25% in those trials that showed greater homocysteine lowering or in persons with no history of stroke. The lowest dose of folic acid required to achieve effective reductions in homocysteine is controversial but important for food fortification policy given recent concerns about the potential adverse effects of overexposure to this vitamin. This study supports the potential benefit of enhancing folate status and/or lowering homocysteine in the primary prevention of stroke. The authors suggest that a folic acid dose as low as 0.2 mg per day can, if administered for 6 months, effectively lower homocysteine concentrations [57].

Numerous studies have shown that a GFD would be sufficient to normalize folate status [21,48,58], but one other [23] show that in a certain percentage of patients, folate levels remain low despite GFD maintained for over 10 years. A possible explanation for this phenomenon is the reduced content of folate in gluten-free foods as previously described by Thompson [49]. Another hypothesis is that in celiac patients genetic alterations of the proteins involved in absorption and metabolism of folate may be present [17].

Hallert et al. suggested providing patients with good information about folate-rich foods. They also recommended starting supplementation in patients who show blood deficiencies after GFD [17,23].

Dosage should be decided in relation to the initial value of the subject. In a study conducted by Hallert et al. on celiac patients, they administered 0.8 mg of folic acid leading to normalization of homocysteine values [24].

In conclusion, folate deficiency was detected in up to 20% of patients on LTGFDWGC. Given this background, a semi-annual routine follow-up of blood folic acid level is mandatory in these subjects. Dosage of supplementation should be decided in relation to the detected value in the subject. The literature suggests supplementation with 1 mg/day of folic acid for 3 months, followed by a reduction to 400–800 mcg/day [30] or with 0.8 mg of folic acid [24] in order to improve the poor folate status.

3.4. Vitamin D and Calcium

This research was carried out based on the keywords "vitamin D" OR "calcium" AND "long-term GFD with good compliance" AND "supplementation" AND "celiac patient" OR "celiac disease". A total of 18 studies were taken into account. Of these studies, 5 were review studies, 4 were prospective studies, 3 were case reports, 2 were observational studies, 2 were guidelines, 1 was a case-control study and 1 was a meta-analysis study.

3.4.1. Vitamin D

The cholecalciferol, or vitamin D3, can be synthesized in the basal layers of the epidermis starting from cholesterol, by the action of ultraviolet rays of sunlight, and this should be the main source of vitamin D for the body. Another source of vitamin D is food, from which the absorption occurs mainly in the terminal ileum.

Numerous studies have shown low levels of vitamin D in many untreated celiac patients. Vitamin D deficiency, investigated through blood value, was detected in about 8–88% of adult CD patients at diagnosis, and in about 0–25% of patients following a GFD [17].

Nevertheless, certain patients, mainly post-menopausal women, continue to present bone density levels below the normal range [59,60]. This seems to be partly due to lack of vitamin D1.

If GFD is not sufficient to bring the values in the normal range, supplementation of vitamin D and calcium is required [17,61–63]. The Endocrine Society guidelines recommend, for the general population, that serum levels of vitamin D are at least equal to 30 ng/mL, and that it is necessary to decide the dosage of supplementation in relation to the initial value of the subject [64].

A meta-analysis conducted on general populations by Shab-Bidar et al. shows that a significant increase in serum levels of vitamin D in adults is achieved with a dose of ≥800 UI/day, at least after 6–12 months of supplementation [65].

Consider that for the celiac patient, a commonly applied strategy in cases of serious vitamin D deficiency is to prescribe a "loading dose" (e.g., 50,000 UI/week for 8 weeks) followed by reduced doses, as shown by Duerksen in a case report study of a woman with CD [66].

In a study aimed at detecting the effects of calcium and vitamin D supplementation in celiac children by Muzzo et al., daily supplementation with 1000 mg of calcium and 400 UI of vitamin D for 24 months was shown to have beneficial effects on the bone mass of celiac patients in whole body and femoral neck measurements; however, these values did not reach the controls [67].

A recent study carried out by Zanchetta et al. suggests an intake of 1000–1500 mg/day of calcium in two or more divided intakes of dairy products and a dose of vitamin D necessary to maintain a blood level of 30 ng/mL [68].

Moreover, Theethira et al. suggested measuring vitamin D levels at diagnosis, repeating every 3 months until levels are normalized, and then every 1–2 years or for symptoms. If necessary, integrate with 1000 (or more-based serum level) UI/day or 50.000 UI weekly if level is <20 ng/mL.

In conclusion, blood vitamin D deficiency was detected in about 0–25% of patients following a LTGFDWGC [69].

3.4.2. Calcium

Calcium deficiency was detected in about 41% of adult patients with CD at the diagnosis [32] and 3.6% of treated children [70]. This seems to be due to malabsorption related to intestinal epithelial damage, but it could also be linked to a reduced expression of a protein regulated by vitamin D that controls the absorption of calcium [17,71]. Calcium absorption is impaired due to mucosal atrophy. Therefore, to avoid hypocalcemia, parathyroid hormone increases substantially (secondary hyperparathyroidism) and stimulates osteoclast-mediated bone degradation. Calcium is then obtained from the skeleton reservoir, but this high remodeling state can lead to osteopenia and osteoporosis, altering bone microstructure and increasing fracture risk [68].

In a study relating to the persistence of calcium deficiency despite a GFD, Kavak et al. undertook the analysis of reduced intake and absorption, rather than the percentage of shortage investigated by blood values in children patients after GFD [70]. The authors reported a reduction in calcium intake in about 76–88% of patients adhering to a GFD [69]. Pazianas et al. described a reduced fractional calcium absorption in adult celiac patients adhering to a GFD despite adequate calcium intake. Taken into account their reduced fractional calcium absorption, the authors concluded that their daily dose should be at least 1200 mg per day [72]. Larussa et al. showed that asymptomatic patients following a GFD for at least 2 years showed normal circulating serum calcium and parathyroid hormone (PTH) levels [73,74]. Zanchetta et al. showed a significant reduction of bone resorption parameters and PTH values, with a significant increase in serum calcium and vitamin D after GFD. Sategna-Guidetti et al.

described significant improvement of bone mineral density values in newly diagnosed CD patients after 1 year of following a GFD [53,68].

Regarding supplementation, Zanchetta et al. suggested 1000–1500 mg/day in two or more divided intakes of dairy products. The authors concluded that calcium supplementation may be an option if the patient is not able or willing to fulfill the required intake through dietary means [68]. Theethira et al. found that more than 50% of patients consume less than the recommended daily intake of calcium. They recommended that CD patients undergo regular assessments with a dietitian and that the recommended intake of calcium, including supplementation should be 1200–1500 mg/day [30].

3.5. Other Micronutrients

This research was carried out based on the keywords "zinc" OR "magnesium" OR "selenium" OR "vitamin K" OR "thiamine" OR "riboflavin" OR "niacin" AND "supplementation" AND "long-term GFD with good compliance" AND "celiac patient" OR "celiac disease". Of the 15 studies that were taken into account, 9 were review studies, 2 were report studies, 2 were prospective studies, 1 was an observational study, and 1 was a case-control study.

3.5.1. Zinc

Zinc deficiency was detected in more than 50% of adult patients with CD at diagnosis, and between 0–40% of patients following a GFD [17]. The lack of this mineral seems to be linked in part to the its reduced absorption, due also to the degree of inflammation of the mucosa.

In the review by Theethira et al., they proposed to measure the serum zinc levels of CD patients at diagnosis and repeat after 3 months until the level is normal, followed by every 1–2 years for symptoms. They also suggested zinc supplementation between 25–40 mg/day until zinc levels were normal [30].

3.5.2. Magnesium

Magnesium deficiency was detected in about 21.4% of adult patients with CD at the diagnosis, and a similar percentage (19.6%) in patients following a GFD [75].

This deficiency can be explained by malabsorption, but GFD may also lead to possible nutrient deficiencies because gluten-free products are usually lower in magnesium, and gluten-free cereals found in nature have a lower magnesium content compared with gluten-containing ones [9].

Furthermore, it has been seen that the resolution of mucosal inflammation may not be sufficient to resolve the shortage of magnesium in celiac patient. The deficiency may also be linked to a reduced intake of this mineral.

Breedon reported that some CD patients need additional magnesium supplement of 200–300 mg/day in the form of magnesium oxide or magnesium chloride, while others can improve magnesium levels through dietary means [76].

3.5.3. Selenium

Selenium deficiency is particularly remarkable because a GFD leads to its absence in cereal foods such as wheat and its derivatives, which are a source of selenium [77]. There are no sufficient literature data to describe a percentage of deficiency investigated through the blood level.

Reduced concentrations of selenium in whole blood, plasma, and leucocytes might develop in several ways. Firstly, GFD might contain a reduced amount of selenium compared with a normal diet, and, secondly, there might be malabsorption of selenium even when the patient is clinically well. Between the extraintestinal symptoms associated with CD, autoimmune thyroid diseases are more evident, underlining that CD-related autoimmune alterations can be modulated not only by gluten but also by various concurrent endogenous (genetic affinity, over-expression of cytokines) and exogenous (environment, nutritional deficiency) factors. The thyroid is particularly sensitive to selenium deficiencies because selenoproteins are significant in biosynthesis and activity of thyroid hormones, while other selenoproteins, including glutathione peroxidase are involved in inhibiting apoptosis. Thus, selenium malabsorption in CD patients can be considered a key factor directly leading to thyroid and intestinal damage [78].

Studies have shown that in celiac patients, selenium supplementation between 120–200 mcg/day is within a safe range. It is important, however, not to exceed the tolerable upper limit of 400 mcg/day for selenium, as this can lead to gastrointestinal upset, hair loss and nerve damage [79].

3.5.4. Vitamin K

Vitamin K deficiency, investigated by markers like PIVKA-II or by prothrombin times, was detected in about 25% of adult patients with CD at the diagnosis, and it seems to return to acceptable levels in almost all patients following a GFD [72,80].

There are limited available data that relate the role of vitamin K and bone health in children and adults with CD. Pazianas et al. examined vitamin K status in children newly diagnosed with CD using prothrombin times as a marker of vitamin K status and found that approximately 35% of children were lacking this marker [72]. However, this may have been an underestimate of the prevalence of vitamin K deficiency as prothrombin time is a very insensitive marker of overall vitamin K status [72]. More sensitive markers of vitamin K status include serum levels of PIVKA-II, which is a vitamin K-dependent protein [80].

In the study carried out by Mager et al., over 25% of children were vitamin K deficient at diagnosis, investigated by PIVKA-II (which is a protein increasing in vitamin K absence), but it resolved in all children after 1 year. This seems to be due in part to improvements in vitamin K intake on the GFD. However, the remaining one-third of children and adolescents continued to have vitamin K intakes considerably lower than the adequate intake on the GFD [80].

Suboptimal dietary intake of vitamin K is common in this population, including when on a GFD. There are no sufficient literature data to recommend a specific dose of supplementation in celiac patient. Therefore, careful consideration should be given to routine supplementation of this nutrient at time of diagnosis of CD.

3.5.5. Niacin, Riboflavin and Thiamin

Deficiency of other micronutrients, like niacin, riboflavin and thiamin have been described in several reviews at the time of diagnosis, although in the literature there is no accurate data on the percentage of celiac patients with such deficiencies [2,16,18]. Deficiencies of niacin and riboflavin may persist after a GFD [2,18]. Regarding thiamin, a study carried out by Shepherd et al. found that the inadequacy of thiamin was more common after GFD implementation than at time of diagnosis [81]. This can be explained by the fact that many gluten-free cereal products do not provide the same levels of thiamin, riboflavin, and/or niacin as enriched wheat flour products. As a result, a GFD that routinely includes gluten-free cereal products could be deficient in one or more of these nutrients, especially if these foods are, in large part, refined and unenriched [82].

Although there is insufficient data in the literature to recommend a dose for supplementation, it is considered useful to carry out control of blood values after diagnosis and after a period of GFD.

4. Discussion

It is evident from the analyzed reviews that there emerges an attention towards nutritional deficiencies that occur in celiac patients after an even longer period of GFD with good compliance. The suggested course of action is a half-yearly routine search in patients on LTGFD nutritional deficiencies, such as low levels of folic acid, vitamin B12, vitamin D, calcium, iron, zinc, selenium and magnesium and the need to establish a personalized supplementation plan, following patients over time, to avoid stopping of integration once the values are returned to their normal range, as shown in Table 2.

Table 2. Supplementation of nutrients in generic state deficiency and in celiac patient.

Nutrient	Route of Administration	Dosage and Sources
Vitamin B12	Oral preferable to intramuscular	• 500 mcg/day ** [24] • 1000 mcg orally until the level is normal and then consider daily gluten-free multi vitamin/mineral supplement ** [30] • 2000 or 1000 mcg/day, then 1000 mcg/week, then 1000 mcg/month * [29]
Iron	Oral preferable to intravenous	• A study on 25 pediatric patients with celiac disease and iron deficiency showed good efficacy of oral administration of iron, (investigated by Bisglycinate Ferrous Chelate) both in patients with gluten-free diet and in those newly diagnosed ** [47] • Therapeutic dose in pediatric patients: 3 mg of elementary iron/kg/day. Prophylactic dose in pediatric patients: 2 mg of elementary iron/kg /day until a maximum dosage of 30 mg/day ** [36] • Iron supplements (325 mg) 1–3 tablets based on initial ferritin level until iron stores are restored. Consider i.v. iron for severe symptomatic iron deficiency anemia or intolerance of oral iron ** [30] • Ferrous sulphate 200 mg 1 or 2/day, (ferrous fumarate, ferrous gluconate) or formulations (iron suspensions) that may also be tolerated better than ferrous sulphate. Oral iron should be continued for 3 months * [46] • Therapy should start with a low dose (one tablet/day of any ferrous sulphate commercially available or any other type of iron), and the intake should be constant until the iron deposits are not restored * [40] • Intravenous ferric carboxymaltose is a stable complex with the advantage of being non-dextran-containing and a very low immunogenic potential and therefore not predisposed to anaphylactic reactions. Its properties permit the administration of large doses (15 mg/kg; maximum of 1000 mg/infusion) in a single and rapid session (15-min infusion) * [45]
Folic acid	Oral preferable to parenteral	• −800 mcg/day ** [24] • 1 mg/day of folic acid for 3 months and once diarrhea improves 400–800 mcg/day ** [30]
Vitamin D—Calcium	Oral preferable to parenteral	• 50.000 U.I./week for 8 weeks, then reduce the dose ** [66] • 1000 mg of calcium and 400 U of vitamin D daily ** [67] • Calcium: 1000–1500 mg/day in two or more divided intakes of dairy products. If the patient is not able or willing to fulfill the required intake through the diet, calcium supplements can be given. Vitamin D: dose necessary to maintain a blood level of 30 ng/mL ** [68] • Vitamin D: 1000 (or more-based serum level) U.I./day or 50.000 U.I. weekly if level is <20 ng/mL. Calcium: recommended intake of calcium, including supplementation, for patients with CD is 1200–1500 mg/day ** [30] • -Vitamin D: ≥800 IU/day, at least for 6/12 months of supplementation * [65]

* Therapy in literature in generic state deficiency ** Therapy in literature in celiac patient.

To help patients reduce deficiencies of minerals (calcium, phosphorus, sodium, potassium, chloride and magnesium) and trace elements (iron, zinc and selenium) it is important to advise them to introduce into their eating habits pseudo-cereals, in which the content of these elements can be twice as high as in other cereals. For example, in teff, iron and calcium contents (11–33 mg/100 g and 100–150 mg/100 g, respectively) are higher than those of wheat, barley, sorghum and rice [18].

It seems important to explain to patients that nutritional education and dietary supplementation should become part of the therapeutic process, which must last a lifetime.

5. Conclusions

In conclusion, if correct GFD is not enough, and the blood levels of micronutrients remain low, it is mandatory to start with personalized supplements. In this case, it would be helpful to evaluate the initial blood level to determine the right dosage of supplementation and repeat the examinations to keep under control values.

In any case, there are a lot of unresolved questions regarding the causes and the mechanisms that lead to these nutritional deficiencies. Further studies are absolutely required for the detailed understanding of this topic.

Supplementary Materials: The following are available online at http://www.mdpi.com/1010-660X/55/7/337/s1, Table S1: Original articles concerning circulating levels and supplementation of micronutrients in celiac patients.

Author Contributions: Conceptualization, M.R.; methodology, S.P.; data curation, G.P., M.A.F., M.N., A.R., M.N. and C.G.; writing—original draft preparation, M.R.; writing—review and editing, T.A.A., S.P. and G.P.

Funding: This research received no external funding.

Conflicts of Interest: The authors declare no conflict of interest.

References

1. Husby, S.; Koletzko, S.; Korponay-Szabó, I.R.; Mearin, M.L.; Phillips, A.; Shamir, R.; Troncone, R.; Giersiepen, K.; Branski, D.; Catassi, C.; et al. European Society for Pediatric Gastroenterology, Hepatology, and Nutrition Guidelines for the Diagnosis of Coeliac Disease. *J. Pediatr. Gastroenterol. Nutr.* **2012**, *54*, 136–160. [CrossRef] [PubMed]
2. Saturni, L.; Ferretti, G.; Bacchetti, T. The Gluten-Free Diet: Safety and Nutritional Quality. *Nutrients* **2010**, *2*, 16–34. [CrossRef] [PubMed]
3. Lindfors, K.; Ciacci, C.; Kurppa, K.; Lundin, K.E.A.; Makharia, G.K.; Mearin, M.L.; Murray, J.A.; Verdu, E.F.; Kaukinen, K. Coeliac Disease. *Nat. Rev. Dis. Primers* **2019**, *5*, 3. [CrossRef] [PubMed]
4. Lebwohl, B.; Sanders, D.S.; Green, P.H.R. Coeliac Disease. *Lancet* **2018**, *391*, 70–81. [CrossRef]
5. De Silvestri, A.; Capittini, C.; Poddighe, D.; Valsecchi, C.; Marseglia, G.; Tagliacarne, S.C.; Scotti, V.; Rebuffi, C.; Pasi, A.; Martinetti, M.; et al. HLA-DQ Genetics in Children with Celiac Disease: A Meta-Analysis Suggesting a Two-Step Genetic Screening Procedure Starting with HLA-DQ β Chains. *Pediatr. Res.* **2018**, *83*, 564–572. [CrossRef] [PubMed]
6. Capittini, C.; De Silvestri, A.; Rebuffi, C.; Tinelli, C.; Poddighe, D.; Capittini, C.; De Silvestri, A.; Rebuffi, C.; Tinelli, C.; Poddighe, D. Relevance of HLA-DQB1*02 Allele in the Genetic Predisposition of Children with Celiac Disease: Additional Cues from a Meta-Analysis. *Medicina (B. Aires)* **2019**, *55*, 190. [CrossRef] [PubMed]
7. Rubio-Tapia, A.; Hill, I.D.; Kelly, C.P.; Calderwood, A.H.; Murray, J.A. ACG Clinical Guidelines: Diagnosis and Management of Celiac Disease. *Am. J. Gastroenterol.* **2013**, *108*, 656–676. [CrossRef]
8. I.C.G.T. *Coeliac Disease*; National Institute for Health and Care Excellence: London, UK, 2015.
9. Vici, G.; Belli, L.; Biondi, M.; Polzonetti, V. Gluten Free Diet and Nutrient Deficiencies: A Review. *Clin. Nutr.* **2016**, *35*, 1236–1241. [CrossRef]
10. Ciacci, C.; Ciclitira, P.; Hadjivassiliou, M.; Kaukinen, K.; Ludvigsson, J.F.; McGough, N.; Sanders, D.S.; Woodward, J.; Leonard, J.N.; Swift, G.L. The Gluten-Free Diet and Its Current Application in Coeliac Disease and Dermatitis Herpetiformis. *United Eur. Gastroenterol. J.* **2015**, *3*, 121–135. [CrossRef]
11. Lanzini, A.; Lanzarotto, F.; Villanacci, V.; Mora, A.; Bertolazzi, S.; Turini, D.; Carella, G.; Malagoli, A.; Ferrante, G.; Cesana, B.M.; et al. Complete Recovery of Intestinal Mucosa Occurs Very Rarely in Adult Coeliac Patients despite Adherence to Gluten-Free Diet. *Aliment. Pharmacol. Ther.* **2009**, *29*, 1299–1308. [CrossRef]
12. Lebwohl, B.; Murray, J.A.; Rubio-Tapia, A.; Green, P.H.R.; Ludvigsson, J.F. Predictors of Persistent Villous Atrophy in Coeliac Disease: A Population-Based Study. *Aliment. Pharmacol. Ther.* **2014**, *39*, 488–495. [CrossRef] [PubMed]
13. Leonard, M.M.; Weir, D.C.; DeGroote, M.; Mitchell, P.D.; Singh, P.; Silvester, J.A.; Leichtner, A.M.; Fasano, A. Value of IgA TTG in Predicting Mucosal Recovery in Children with Celiac Disease on a Gluten-Free Diet. *J. Pediatr. Gastroenterol. Nutr.* **2017**, *64*, 286–291. [CrossRef] [PubMed]
14. Kaukinen, K.; Peraaho, M.; Lindfors, K.; Partanen, J.; Woolley, N.; Pikkarainen, P.; Karvonen, A.-L.; Laasanen, T.; Sievaneh, H.; Maki, M.; et al. Persistent Small Bowel Mucosal Villous Atrophy without Symptoms in Coeliac Disease. *Aliment. Pharmacol. Ther.* **2007**, *25*, 1237–1245. [CrossRef]

15. Egger, M.; Dickersin, K.; Smith, G.D. Problems and Limitations in Conducting Systematic Reviews. In *Systematic Reviews in Health Care*; BMJ Publishing Group: London, UK, 2008; pp. 43–68.
16. Kupper, C. Dietary Guidelines and Implementation for Celiac Disease. *Gastroenterology* **2005**, *128* (Suppl. 1), S121–S127. [CrossRef]
17. Caruso, R.; Pallone, F.; Stasi, E.; Romeo, S.; Monteleone, G. Appropriate Nutrient Supplementation in Celiac Disease. *Ann. Med.* **2013**, *45*, 522–531. [CrossRef]
18. Penagini, F.; Dilillo, D.; Meneghin, F.; Mameli, C.; Fabiano, V.; Zuccotti, G.V. Gluten-Free Diet in Children: An Approach to a Nutritionally Adequate and Balanced Diet. *Nutrients* **2013**, *5*, 4553–4565. [CrossRef]
19. Harper, J.W.; Holleran, S.F.; Ramakrishnan, R.; Bhagat, G.; Green, P.H.R. Anemia in Celiac Disease Is Multifactorial in Etiology. *Am. J. Hematol.* **2007**, *82*, 996–1000. [CrossRef] [PubMed]
20. Dahele, A.; Ghosh, S. Vitamin B12 Deficiency in Untreated Celiac Disease. *Am. J. Gastroenterol.* **2001**, *96*, 745–750. [CrossRef]
21. Dickey, W.; Ward, M.; Whittle, C.R.; Kelly, M.T.; Pentieva, K.; Horigan, G.; Patton, S.; McNulty, H. Homocysteine and Related B-Vitamin Status in Coeliac Disease: Effects of Gluten Exclusion and Histological Recovery. *Scand. J. Gastroenterol.* **2008**, *43*, 682–688. [CrossRef]
22. Halfdanarson, T.R.; Litzow, M.R.; Murray, J.A. Hematologic Manifestations of Celiac Disease. *Blood* **2007**, *109*, 412–421. [CrossRef]
23. Hallert, C.; Grant, C.; Grehn, S.; Grännö, C.; Hultén, S.; Midhagen, G.; Ström, M.; Svensson, H.; Valdimarsson, T. Evidence of Poor Vitamin Status in Coeliac Patients on a Gluten-Free Diet for 10 Years. *Aliment. Pharmacol. Ther.* **2002**, *16*, 1333–1339. [CrossRef] [PubMed]
24. Hallert, C.; Svensson, M.; Tholstrup, J.; Hultberg, B. Clinical Trial: B Vitamins Improve Health in Patients with Coeliac Disease Living on a Gluten-Free Diet. *Aliment. Pharmacol. Ther.* **2009**, *29*, 811–816. [CrossRef] [PubMed]
25. Green, R. Indicators for Assessing Folate and Vitamin B-12 Status and for Monitoring the Efficacy of Intervention Strategies. *Am. J. Clin. Nutr.* **2011**, *94*, 666S–672S. [CrossRef] [PubMed]
26. Ludvigsson, J.F.; Welander, A.; Lassila, R.; Ekbom, A.; Montgomery, S.M. Risk of Thromboembolism in 14,000 Individuals with Coeliac Disease. *Br. J. Haematol.* **2007**, *139*, 121–127. [CrossRef] [PubMed]
27. Eichinger, S. Are B Vitamins a Risk Factor for Venous Thromboembolism? Yes. *J. Thromb. Haemost.* **2006**, *4*, 307–308. [CrossRef] [PubMed]
28. Bolaman, Z.; Kadikoylu, G.; Yukselen, V.; Yavasoglu, I.; Barutca, S.; Senturk, T. Oral versus Intramuscular Cobalamin Treatment in Megaloblastic Anemia: A Single-Center, Prospective, Randomized, Open-Label Study. *Clin Ther.* **2003**, *25*, 3124–3134. [CrossRef]
29. Vidal-Alaball, J.; Butler, C.C.; Cannings-John, R.; Goringe, A.; Hood, K.; McCaddon, A.; McDowell, I.; Papaioannou, A. Oral Vitamin B12 versus Intramuscular Vitamin B12 for Vitamin B12 Deficiency. *Cochrane Database Syst. Rev.* **2005**, *3*. [CrossRef] [PubMed]
30. Theethira, T.G.; Dennis, M.; Leffler, D.A. Nutritional Consequences of Celiac Disease and the Gluten-Free Diet. *Expert Rev. Gastroenterol. Hepatol.* **2014**, *8*, 123–129. [CrossRef]
31. Fasano, A.; Berti, I.; Gerarduzzi, T.; Not, T.; Colletti, R.B.; Drago, S.; Elitsur, Y.; Green, P.H.R.; Guandalini, S.; Hill, I.D.; et al. Prevalence of Celiac Disease in At-Risk and Not-at-Risk Groups in the United States: A Large Multicenter Study. *Arch. Intern. Med.* **2003**, *163*, 286–292. [CrossRef]
32. Malterre, T. Digestive and Nutritional Considerations in Celiac Disease: Could Supplementation Help? *Altern. Med. Rev.* **2009**, *14*, 247–257.
33. Haapalahti, M.; Kulmala, P.; Karttunen, T.J.; Paajanen, L.; Laurila, K.; Mäki, M.; Mykkänen, H.; Kokkonen, J. Nutritional Status in Adolescents and Young Adults with Screen-Detected Celiac Disease. *J. Pediatr. Gastroenterol. Nutr.* **2005**, *40*, 566–570. [CrossRef] [PubMed]
34. Lo, W.; Sano, K.; Lebwohl, B.; Diamond, B.; Green, P.H.R. Changing Presentation of Adult Celiac Disease. *Dig. Dis. Sci.* **2003**, *48*, 395–398. [CrossRef] [PubMed]
35. Kolho, K.L.; Färkkilä, M.A.; Savilahti, E. Undiagnosed Coeliac Disease Is Common in Finnish Adults. *Scand. J. Gastroenterol.* **1998**, *33*, 1280–1283. [PubMed]
36. Kapur, G.; Patwari, A.K.; Narayan, S.; Anand, V.K. Iron Supplementation in Children with Celiac Disease. *Indian J. Pediatr.* **2003**, *70*, 955–958. [CrossRef] [PubMed]

37. Annibale, B.; Severi, C.; Chistolini, A.; Antonelli, G.; Lahner, E.; Marcheggiano, A.; Iannoni, C.; Monarca, B.; Delle Fave, G. Efficacy of Gluten-Free Diet Alone on Recovery from Iron Deficiency Anemia in Adult Celiac Patients. *Am. J. Gastroenterol.* **2001**, *96*, 132–137. [CrossRef]
38. Hopper, A.D.; Leeds, J.S.; Hurlstone, D.P.; Hadjivassiliou, M.; Drew, K.; Sanders, D.S. Are Lower Gastrointestinal Investigations Necessary in Patients with Coeliac Disease? *Eur. J. Gastroenterol. Hepatol.* **2005**, *17*, 617–621. [CrossRef]
39. Oxford, E.C.; Nguyen, D.D.; Sauk, J.; Korzenik, J.R.; Yajnik, V.; Friedman, S.; Ananthakrishnan, A.N. Impact of Coexistent Celiac Disease on Phenotype and Natural History of Inflammatory Bowel Diseases. *Am. J. Gastroenterol.* **2013**, *108*, 1123–1129. [CrossRef]
40. Aspuru, K.; Villa, C.; Bermejo, F.; Herrero, P.; López, S.G. Optimal Management of Iron Deficiency Anemia Due to Poor Dietary Intake. *Int. J. Gen. Med.* **2011**, *4*, 741–750. [CrossRef]
41. Mimura, E.C.M.; Breganó, J.W.; Dichi, J.B.; Gregório, E.P.; Dichi, I. Comparison of Ferrous Sulfate and Ferrous Glycinate Chelate for the Treatment of Iron Deficiency Anemia in Gastrectomized Patients. *Nutrition* **2008**, *24*, 663–668. [CrossRef]
42. Pineda, O.; Ashmead, H.D. Effectiveness of Treatment of Iron-Deficiency Anemia in Infants and Young Children with Ferrous Bis-Glycinate Chelate. *Nutrition* **2001**, *17*, 381–384. [CrossRef]
43. Fishbane, S.; Kowalski, E.A. The Comparative Safety of Intravenous Iron Dextran, Iron Saccharate, and Sodium Ferric Gluconate. *Semin. Dial.* **2000**, *13*, 381–384. [CrossRef] [PubMed]
44. Kulnigg, S.; Stoinov, S.; Simanenkov, V.; Dudar, L.V.; Karnafel, W.; Garcia, L.C.; Sambuelli, A.M.; D'Haens, G.; Gasche, C. A Novel Intravenous Iron Formulation for Treatment of Anemia in Inflammatory Bowel Disease: The Ferric Carboxymaltose (FERINJECT) Randomized Controlled Trial. *Am. J. Gastroenterol.* **2008**, *103*, 1182–1192. [CrossRef] [PubMed]
45. Friedrisch, J.R.; Cançado, R.D. Intravenous Ferric Carboxymaltose for the Treatment of Iron Deficiency Anemia. *Rev. Bras. Hematol. Hemoter.* **2015**, *37*, 400–405. [CrossRef] [PubMed]
46. Goddard, A.F.; McIntyre, A.S.; Scott, B.B. Guidelines for the Management of Iron Deficiency Anaemia. British Society of Gastroenterology. *Gut* **2000**, *46* (Suppl. 3–4), IV1–IV5. [CrossRef] [PubMed]
47. Mazza, G.A.; Marrazzo, S.; Gangemi, P.; Battaglia, E.; Giancotti, L.; Miniero, R. Oral Iron Absorption Test with Ferrous Bisglycinate Chelate in Children with Celiac Disease. *Minerva Pediatr.* **2019**, *71*, 139–143. [CrossRef] [PubMed]
48. Vilppula, A.; Kaukinen, K.; Luostarinen, L.; Krekelä, I.; Patrikainen, H.; Valve, R.; Luostarinen, M.; Laurila, K.; Mäki, M.; Collin, P. Clinical Benefit of Gluten-Free Diet in Screen-Detected Older Celiac Disease Patients. *BMC Gastroenterol.* **2011**, *11*, 136. [CrossRef] [PubMed]
49. Thompson, T. Folate, Iron, and Dietary Fiber Contents of the Gluten-Free Diet. *J. Am. Diet. Assoc.* **2000**, *100*, 1389–1396. [CrossRef]
50. Centers for Disease Control and Prevention (CDC). Trends in Wheat-Flour Fortification with Folic Acid and Iron–Worldwide, 2004 and 2007. *MMWR. Morb. Mortal. Wkly. Rep.* **2008**, *57*, 8–10.
51. Howard, M.R.; Turnbull, A.J.; Morley, P.; Hollier, P.; Webb, R.; Clarke, A. A Prospective Study of the Prevalence of Undiagnosed Coeliac Disease in Laboratory Defined Iron and Folate Deficiency. *J. Clin. Pathol.* **2002**, *55*, 754–757. [CrossRef]
52. Hallert, C.; Tobiasson, P.; Walan, A. Serum Folate Determinations in Tracing Adult Coeliacs. *Scand. J. Gastroenterol.* **1981**, *16*, 263–267. [CrossRef]
53. Sategna-Guidetti, C.; Grosso, S.B.; Grosso, S.; Mengozzi, G.; Aimo, G.; Zaccaria, T.; Di Stefano, M.; Isaia, G.C. The Effects of 1-Year Gluten Withdrawal on Bone Mass, Bone Metabolism and Nutritional Status in Newly-Diagnosed Adult Coeliac Disease Patients. *Aliment. Pharmacol. Ther.* **2000**, *14*, 35–43. [CrossRef]
54. Ponziani, F.R.; Cazzato, I.A.; Danese, S.; Fagiuoli, S.; Gionchetti, P.; Annicchiarico, B.E.; D'Aversa, F.; Gasbarrini, A. Folate in Gastrointestinal Health and Disease. *Eur. Rev. Med. Pharmacol. Sci.* **2012**, *16*, 376–385. [PubMed]
55. Patwari, A.K.; Anand, V.K.; Kapur, G.; Narayan, S. Clinical and Nutritional Profile of Children with Celiac Disease. *Indian Pediatr.* **2003**, *40*, 337–342. [PubMed]
56. Kemppainen, T.A.; Kosma, V.M.; Janatuinen, E.K.; Julkunen, R.J.; Pikkarainen, P.H.; Uusitupa, M.I. Nutritional Status of Newly Diagnosed Celiac Disease Patients before and after the Institution of a Celiac Disease Diet–Association with the Grade of Mucosal Villous Atrophy. *Am. J. Clin. Nutr.* **1998**, *67*, 482–487. [CrossRef] [PubMed]

57. Tighe, P.; Ward, M.; McNulty, H.; Finnegan, O.; Dunne, A.; Strain, J.; Molloy, A.M.; Duffy, M.; Pentieva, K.; Scott, J.M. A Dose-Finding Trial of the Effect of Long-Term Folic Acid Intervention: Implications for Food Fortification Policy. *Am. J. Clin. Nutr.* **2011**, *93*, 11–18. [CrossRef] [PubMed]
58. Saibeni, S.; Lecchi, A.; Meucci, G.; Cattaneo, M.; Tagliabue, L.; Rondonotti, E.; Formenti, S.; De Franchis, R.; Vecchi, M. Prevalence of Hyperhomocysteinemia in Adult Gluten-Sensitive Enteropathy at Diagnosis: Role of B12, Folate, and Genetics. *Clin. Gastroenterol. Hepatol.* **2005**, *3*, 574–580. [CrossRef]
59. Pantaleoni, S.; Luchino, M.; Adriani, A.; Pellicano, R.; Stradella, D.; Ribaldone, D.G.; Sapone, N.; Isaia, G.C.; Di Stefano, M.; Astegiano, M. Bone Mineral Density at Diagnosis of Celiac Disease and after 1 Year of Gluten-Free Diet. *Sci. World J.* **2014**, *2014*, 1–6. [CrossRef]
60. Szymczak, J.; Bohdanowicz-Pawlak, A.; Waszczuk, E.; Jakubowska, J. Low Bone Mineral Density in Adult Patients with Coeliac Disease. *Endokrynol. Pol.* **2012**, *63*, 270–276. [CrossRef]
61. García-Porrúa, C.; González-Gay, M.A.; Avila-Alvarenga, S.; Rivas, M.J.; Soilan, J.; Penedo, M. Coeliac Disease and Osteomalacia: An Association Still Present in Western Countries. *Rheumatology* **2000**, *39*, 1435. [CrossRef]
62. McNicholas, B.A.; Bell, M. Coeliac Disease Causing Symptomatic Hypocalcaemia, Osteomalacia and Coagulapathy. *BMJ Case Rep.* **2010**, *2010*, bcr0920092262. [CrossRef]
63. Sahebari, M.; Sigari, S.Y.; Heidari, H.; Biglarian, O. Osteomalacia Can Still Be a Point of Attention to Celiac Disease. *Clin. Cases Miner. Bone Metab.* **2011**, *8*, 14–15. [PubMed]
64. Holick, M.F.; Binkley, N.C.; Bischoff-Ferrari, H.A.; Gordon, C.M.; Hanley, D.A.; Heaney, R.P.; Murad, M.H.; Weaver, C.M.; Endocrine Society. Evaluation, Treatment, and Prevention of Vitamin D Deficiency: An Endocrine Society Clinical Practice Guideline. *J. Clin. Endocrinol. Metab.* **2011**, *96*, 1911–1930. [CrossRef] [PubMed]
65. Shab-Bidar, S.; Bours, S.; Geusens, P.P.M.M.; Kessels, A.G.H.; van den Bergh, J.P.W. Serum 25(OH)D Response to Vitamin D3 Supplementation: A Meta-Regression Analysis. *Nutrition* **2014**, *30*, 975–985. [CrossRef] [PubMed]
66. Duerksen, D.R.; Ali, M.; Leslie, W.D. Dramatic Effect of Vitamin D Supplementation and a Gluten-Free Diet on Bone Mineral Density in a Patient with Celiac Disease. *J. Clin. Densitom.* **2012**, *15*, 120–123. [CrossRef]
67. Muzzo, S.; Burrows, R.; Burgueño, M.; Ríos, G.; Bergenfreid, C.; Chavez, E.; Leiva, L. Effect of Calcium and Vitamin D Supplementation on Bone Mineral Density of Celiac Children. *Nutr. Res.* **2000**, *20*, 1241–1247. [CrossRef]
68. Zanchetta, M.B.; Longobardi, V.; Bai, J.C. Bone and Celiac Disease. *Curr. Osteoporos. Rep.* **2016**, *14*, 43–48. [CrossRef] [PubMed]
69. Krupa-Kozak, U. Pathologic Bone Alterations in Celiac Disease: Etiology, Epidemiology, and Treatment. *Nutrition* **2014**, *30*, 16–24. [CrossRef] [PubMed]
70. Kavak, U.S.; Yüce, A.; Kocak, N.; Demir, H.; Saltik, I.N.; Gürakan, F.; Ozen, H. Bone Mineral Density in Children with Untreated and Treated Celiac Disease. *J. Pediatr. Gastroenterol. Nutr.* **2003**, *37*, 434–436. [CrossRef] [PubMed]
71. Staun, M.; Jarnum, S. Measurement of the 10,000-Molecular Weight Calcium-Binding Protein in Small-Intestinal Biopsy Specimens from Patients with Malabsorption Syndromes. *Scand. J. Gastroenterol.* **1988**, *23*, 827–832. [CrossRef]
72. Pazianas, M.; Butcher, G.P.; Subhani, J.M.; Finch, P.J.; Ang, L.; Collins, C.; Heaney, R.P.; Zaidi, M.; Maxwell, J.D. Calcium Absorption and Bone Mineral Density in Celiacs after Long Term Treatment with Gluten-Free Diet and Adequate Calcium Intake. *Osteoporos. Int.* **2005**, *16*, 56–63. [CrossRef]
73. Larussa, T.; Suraci, E.; Nazionale, I.; Leone, I.; Montalcini, T.; Abenavoli, L.; Imeneo, M.; Pujia, A.; Luzza, F. No Evidence of Circulating Autoantibodies against Osteoprotegerin in Patients with Celiac Disease. *World J. Gastroenterol.* **2012**, *18*, 1622–1627. [CrossRef] [PubMed]
74. Larussa, T.; Suraci, E.; Imeneo, M.; Marasco, R.; Luzza, F. Normal Bone Mineral Density Associates with Duodenal Mucosa Healing in Adult Patients with Celiac Disease on a Gluten-Free Diet. *Nutrients* **2017**, *9*, 98. [CrossRef] [PubMed]
75. Rujner, J.; Socha, J.; Syczewska, M.; Wojtasik, A.; Kunachowicz, H.; Stolarczyk, A. Magnesium Status in Children and Adolescents with Coeliac Disease without Malabsorption Symptoms. *Clin. Nutr.* **2004**, *23*, 1074–1079. [CrossRef] [PubMed]

76. Breedon, C. Medical Center Aunt Cathy's Guide to: Thinking About OTHER Nutrition Issues in Celiac Disease. Available online: http://www.mnsna.org/wp-content/uploads/2010/07/Aunt-C-Celiac-Disease-short-OtherNutr-Issues-Sanf-this-12-no-date.pdf (accessed on 3 July 2019).
77. Stazi, A.V.; Trinti, B. Selenium Status and Over-Expression of Interleukin-15 in Celiac Disease and Autoimmune Thyroid Diseases. *Ann. Ist. Super. Sanita* **2010**, *46*, 389–399. [CrossRef] [PubMed]
78. Hinks, L.J.; Inwards, K.D.; Lloyd, B.; Clayton, B.E. Body Content of Selenium in Coeliac Disease. *Br. Med. J.* **1984**, *288*, 1862–1863. [CrossRef]
79. Faerber Emily Community Rotation. Selenium Supplement Information for Your Gluten-Free Patients. 2011. Available online: http://depts.washington.edu/nutr/wordpress/wp-content/uploads/2015/03/Selenium_2012.pdf (accessed on 3 July 2019).
80. Mager, D.R.; Qiao, J.; Turner, J. Vitamin D and K Status Influences Bone Mineral Density and Bone Accrual in Children and Adolescents with Celiac Disease. *Eur. J. Clin. Nutr.* **2012**, *66*, 488–495. [CrossRef]
81. Shepherd, S.J.; Gibson, P.R. Nutritional Inadequacies of the Gluten-Free Diet in Both Recently-Diagnosed and Long-Term Patients with Coeliac Disease. *J. Hum. Nutr. Diet.* **2013**, *26*, 349–358. [CrossRef]
82. Thompson, T. Thiamin, Riboflavin, and Niacin Contents of the Gluten-Free Diet: Is There Cause for Concern? *J. Am. Diet. Assoc.* **1999**, *99*, 858–862. [CrossRef]

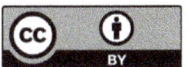

© 2019 by the authors. Licensee MDPI, Basel, Switzerland. This article is an open access article distributed under the terms and conditions of the Creative Commons Attribution (CC BY) license (http://creativecommons.org/licenses/by/4.0/).

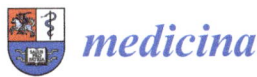

Review

Non-Celiac Gluten Sensitivity: A Review

Anna Roszkowska [1,*], Marta Pawlicka [1], Anna Mroczek [1], Kamil Bałabuszek [1] and Barbara Nieradko-Iwanicka [2]

1. Medical University of Lublin, Radziwillowska 11 Street, 20-080 Lublin, Poland; martamisztal991@gmail.com (M.P.); anna.mroczek94@wp.pl (A.M.); balkam@o2.pl (K.B.)
2. Chair and Department of Hygiene, Medical University of Lublin, Radziwillowska 11 Street, 20-080 Lublin, Poland; barbaranieradkoiwanicka@umlub.pl
* Correspondence: annros7@gmail.com

Received: 2 February 2019; Accepted: 22 May 2019; Published: 28 May 2019

Abstract: *Background and objectives:* Grain food consumption is a trigger of gluten related disorders: celiac disease, non-celiac gluten sensitivity (NCGS) and wheat allergy. They demonstrate with non-specific symptoms: bloating, abdominal discomfort, diarrhea and flatulence. Aim: The aim of the review is to summarize data about pathogenesis, symptoms and criteria of NCGS, which can be helpful for physicians. *Materials and Methods:* The PubMed and Google Scholar databases were searched in January 2019 with phrases: 'non-celiac gluten sensitivity', non-celiac gluten sensitivity', non-celiac wheat gluten sensitivity', non-celiac wheat gluten sensitivity', and gluten sensitivity'. More than 1000 results were found. A total of 67 clinical trials published between 1989 and 2019 was scanned. After skimming abstracts, 66 articles were chosen for this review; including 26 clinical trials. *Results:* In 2015, Salerno Experts' Criteria of NCGS were published. The Salerno first step is assessing the clinical response to gluten free diet (GFD) and second is measuring the effect of reintroducing gluten after a period of treatment with GFD. Several clinical trials were based on the criteria. *Conclusions:* Symptoms of NCGS are similar to other gluten-related diseases, irritable bowel syndrome and Crohn's disease. With Salerno Experts' Criteria of NCGS, it is possible to diagnose patients properly and give them advice about nutritional treatment.

Keywords: non-celiac gluten sensitivity; irritable bowel disease; gluten; FODMAP; wheat allergy

1. Introduction

Wheat, rice and maize are the most commonly consumed grains worldwide. These products are rich sources of starch—the basic dietary component for the growing human population [1]. Wheat contains gluten. In 1953 Dickie, van de Kamer and Weyers published a study confirming malabsorption after wheat consumption in patients with celiac disease (CD) [2]. Nowadays, gluten intake is considered to be the trigger of gluten related disorders (GRDs). In GRD, the gluten-free diet (GFD) is principal, effective and yet the only treatment method. The gluten-free market is still rising, not only because of growing interest and public awareness of GRDs, but also due to celebrities touting this diet by for weight loss and athletes for improved performance [3], which is debatable as grains should be the main source of energy in the human diet.

2. Materials and Methods

Standard up-to-date criteria were followed for review of the literature data. A search for English-language articles in the PubMed database was performed. The PubMed and Google Scholar databases were searched in January 2019 with phrases: 'non-celiac gluten sensitivity', non-celiac gluten sensitivity', non-celiac wheat gluten sensitivity', non-celiac wheat gluten sensitivity', and gluten sensitivity'. More than 1000 results were found. A total of 67 clinical trials published between 1989 and 2019 was scanned. After skimming abstracts, 66 articles were chosen for this review including 26 clinical trials.

2.1. Gluten Related Disorders (GRDs)

The term "gluten intolerance" includes three different conditions: CD, allergy to wheat (WA) and non-celiac gluten sensitivity (NCGS) [4]. To date, CD and WA comprise for the best known and studied entities, which are mediated by immune system [1]. WA—classified as a classic food allergy is induced by wheat (not only gluten) intake that leads to type I and type IV hypersensitivity. The crucial role in WA disorder play IgE immunoglobulins [1,5]. CD is an autoimmune disease occurring in genetically susceptible individuals with HLA-DQ2 and/or HLA-DQ8 genotypes. CD is characterized by the presence of specific serological antibodies such as: anti-tissue transglutaminase (tTG) IgA, anti-endomysium IgA (EMA) and anti-deamidated gliadin peptides IgG (DPG) [1]. There were reported cases of patients with gluten sensitivity in which allergic and autoimmune mechanisms could not be identified. They were collectively described as NCGS [1]. The NCGS or "non-celiac wheat sensitivity" (NCWS) has been a topic of interest in recent years. This trend is associated with a large number of studies concerning the syndrome [6,7]. The term NCWS is more adequate because of components other than gluten, that may contribute to intestinal and extra-intestinal symptoms [6]. In 1980, Cooper et al. described intestinal gluten-sensitive symptoms in 8 patients in whom CD was ruled out [8]. Further studies led to the definition of NCGS. NCGS is a condition characterized by clinical and pathological manifestations, related to gluten ingestion in individuals in whom CD and WA have been excluded [1,6,9,10]. Leccioli et al. described NCGS as a multi-factor-onset disorder, perhaps temporary and preventable, associated with an unbalanced diet [11].

Interestingly, II MHC haplotype HLA-DQ2 and HLA-DQ8 typical for CD is present only in about 50% of NCGS patients [1]. The main features of GRDs are summarized in Table 1.

Table 1. Comparison of prevalence, pathogenic, and diagnostic features of gluten related disorders (GRDs); non-celiac gluten sensitivity (NCGS), IgA anti-EMA (IgA antibodies against endomysium), IgA anti-tTG (IgA antibodies against transglutaminase), IgG anti-DGP (IgG antibodies against deamidated gliadin peptides).

	Celiac Disease	NCGS	Wheat Allergy
Prevalence	0.5–1.7%	no population studies	0.5–9% in children
Pathogenesis	autoimmune	non-specific immune response	IgE mediated response
DQ2-DQ8 HLA haplotypes	positive in 95% cases	positive in 50% cases	negative
Serological markers	IgA anti-EMA, IgA anti-tTG, IgG anti-DGP, IgA anti-gliadin	IgA/IgG anti-gliadin in 50% cases	specific IgE antibodies against wheat and gliadin
Duodenal biopsy *	Marsh I to IV with domination of Marsh III and IV	Marsh 0-II, but according to some experts Marsh III might also be in NCGS	Marsh 0-II
Duodenal villi atrophy	present	absent	might be present or absent

* Marsh classification.

2.2. Epidemiology of Gluten Related Disorders (GRDs)

CD morbidity, based on serological results, is estimated to be 1.1% to 1.7% worldwide [12,13]. WA among children occurs with a frequency of 0.4–9% [5,14]. Due to an absence of diagnostic markers and population studies, the prevalence of NCGS is not well established [5,6]. Although studies have been conducted by several authors, this problem is still insufficiently explored. Previous data were based primarily on questionnaires for self-reported gluten sensitivity SR-GS/self-reported NCGS. According to several authors, the NCGS prevalence is from 0.6% up to 13% of the general population [15–19]. NCGS was reported more often among women [16–18], adults in the fourth decade of life [19,20] and individuals coming from urban area [18]. Among intestinal symptoms the most frequent in NCGS are: bloating, abdominal discomfort and pain, diarrhea and flatulence.

The most common extra-intestinal symptoms were: tiredness, headache and anxiety [15,16,18,20]. Differentiation between NCGS and functional gastrointestinal (GI) disease—mainly irritable bowel syndrome (IBS)—may be difficult as some of the above-mentioned symptoms overlap with IBS manifestations. Van Gils et al. pointed that 37% of self-reported gluten sensitivity individuals (SR-GS) fulfilled the Rome III criteria for IBS, in contrast to 9% prevalence in the control group [18]. Similar findings were reported by Carroccio et al. IBS symptoms were reported in 44% self-reported NCWS [15]. According to research conducted by Cabrera et al., IBS, eating disorders and lactose intolerance were present more often in SR-GS individuals than in non-SR-GS group (14.3% vs. 4.7%) [16]. Herein, discussed studies indicate that SR-GS/SR-NCGS may correlate with more frequent occurrence of IBS, comparing to the general population. However, the German Society of Allergology and Clinical Immunology emphasized that the publications about NCGS suffer from certain weaknesses: absence of validated diagnostic criteria, suitable biomarkers, frequent self-diagnosis and unconfirmed etiology of reported symptoms. Thus, the prevalence of NCGS cannot be clearly established [21].

2.3. Gluten

Gluten is defined as a family of proteins found in grains (wheat, rye, barley, oats). It includes two main proteins: gliadin and glutenin. Also, similar proteins such as secalin in rye, harden in barley and avenues in oats contribute to the definition of 'gluten' [22]. Gluten proteins are characterized by high proline and glutamine content, moreover, they are resistant to proteolytic enzymes in the gastrointestinal tract. In some individuals these peptides can cross the epithelial barrier and activate immune system: trigger an allergic (WA) or autoimmune response (CD) [5]. Incomplete digestion leads to significant changes in human gut and causes intestinal or extra-intestinal symptoms. Gliadin and other gluten proteins stimulate T-cells. Some authors suggested that amylase-tripsin inhibitors (ATIs) and fermentable oligo-, di-, and mono-saccharides and polyols (FODMAPs) may be associated with NCGS [11]. Another wheat constituent, known as agglutinin-carbohydrate binding protein and exorphins seem to influence immune system and induce damage of intestinal epithelium [11,22].

2.4. Amylase-Tripsin Inhibitors (ATIs)

ATIs are albumin proteins found in wheat representing up to 4% of total proteins in grains [1]. They are highly resistant to intestinal proteases [1] and may induce release of pro-inflammatory cytokines from monocytes, macrophages and dendritic cells through activation of a toll-like receptor-4 in CD and NCGS patients [1,22]. ATIs may provoke activation of innate immune cells and intestinal inflammation [21]. ATIs activate immunological system through effect on toll-like receptor-4 in CD, that was confirmed in the research conducted by Junker et al. on mice deficient in TLR4 or TLR signaling [23]. Authors observed, that their mice models were protected from intestinal and systemic immune responses during oral ATIs intake [23]. Scientists also confirmed, that ATIs stimulate monocytes, macrophages and dendritic cells *in vitro* to produce IL-8, IL-12, TNF, MCP-1 and Regulated on Activation, Normal T-cell Expressed and Secreted (RANTES) [23].

2.5. Fermentable Oligo-, Di- and Mono-Saccharides and Polyols (FODMAPs)

FODMAPs are short-chain sugars with less than 10 carbon atoms in the molecule [24]. The attention of scientists in recent years was drawn to the potential contribution of FODMAPS to pathogenesis of gastrointestinal disorders [25]. The scientists from Monash University in Australia conducted thorough analysis of a group of carbohydrates, which, despite their different structures, produced similar postprandial effects. The most prevalent forms of FODMAP include: fructooligosaccharides (FOS), galactooligosaccharides (GOS), lactose, fructose, polyols, sorbitol and mannitol. Barrett et al. created a list of food products that are good sources of FODMAP (Figure 1) and poor in short chain sugars (Figure 2) [24].

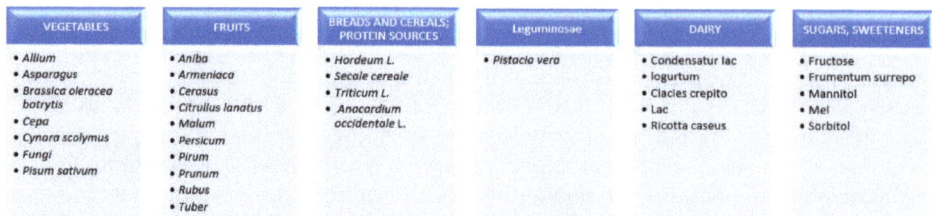

Figure 1. List of products being the source of fermentable oligo-, di-, and mono-saccharides and polyols (FODMAPs).

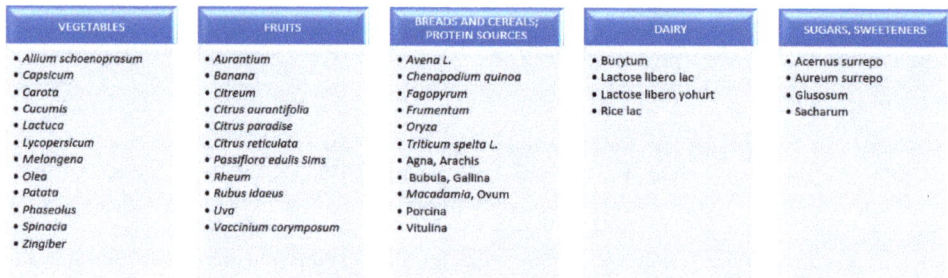

Figure 2. List of products low in FODMAPs.

Compounds belonging to the FODMAP group are not digested nor absorbed in the gastrointestinal tract. They have a strong osmotic effect and undergo rapid fermentation in the intestines, resulting in intestinal liquefaction, excessive gas production, bloating and pain. They may cause or exacerbate symptoms in susceptible patients with inflammatory bowel disease and irritable bowel syndrome (IBS) [24,25]. Numerous studies have confirmed the improvement in patients suffering from ulcerative colitis, Crohn's Disease and IBS following the elimination of short-chain sugars from the diet [26].

Wheat is a rich source of gluten and also contains large amounts of FODMAPs, which play a key role in NCGS development [27]. Some researchers suggest that diet low in FODMAP is beneficial for NCGS patients [25].

Considering the above research results, scientists are leaning towards renaming NCGS to a more recent NCWS [27]. It should be emphasized that a diet poor in FODMAPs should not be used without medical indications, as healthy people do not benefit from such diet [24]. Moreover, it was proven that FOS and GOS, compounds belonging to FODMAPS, alike prebiotic, favor proper colonization of intestines with *Bifidobacteria* and *Lactobacilli* bacteria and limit the proliferation of *Bacteroides* spp., *Clostridium* spp. and *Escherichia coli*. There is evidence that short-chain fatty acids (SCFA)—the product of FODMAP fermentation—have protective properties against colorectal cancer [24,27]. FODMAPs are believed to have a positive effect on lipid metabolism by lowering serum cholesterol, triglycerides and phospholipids [27]. In addition, this diet leads to calcium absorption disorders, lowering its serum levels. People resigning from products that are the source of FODMAP are at risk of vitamin and antioxidants deficiency [27,28]. Therefore, it is suggested to supplement vitamins, pro- and prebiotics when switching to the low FODMAPs diet [24,27].

2.6. The Salerno Experts' Criteria of NCGS

As long as the NCGS biomarker is not available, certain limitations are included in two-step diagnostic protocol introduced in 2015. However, up to date The Salerno Experts' Criteria constitute the only accessible recommendations for diagnosis of NCGS. It should be emphasized that according to currently used criteria, NCGS should not be based only on exclusion diagnosis, which is new in comparison to the former practice [29]. Thus, the guidelines indicate the need of a standardized procedure: 6-week course of gluten-free diet—with the simultaneous, continuous assessment of symptoms and their intensity, followed by measuring the effect of reintroducing gluten after a period of treatment with GFD. A modified version of the Gastrointestinal Symptom Rating Scale (GSRS) was found to be applicable in terms of symptoms evaluation. Although limited, double-blind-placebo-controlled (DBPC) procedure remains to be the golden standard in NCGS investigation, yet, single-blinded procedure is allowed for the purposes of clinical practice [29–31]. The guidelines stress the importance of patient compliance, especially when it comes to shift to GFD, which should be discussed with a dietitian before implementation [29].

Back to the limitations—it is recommended to use gluten in the form of commonly consumed food products, during gluten challenge, rather than in the form of gluten capsules. Nevertheless, there is presumption that ATIs and FODMAPS—as the constituents of grains—interfere with the DPBC results [6,30,32]. Moreover, since the study on patients complaining about IBS-like symptoms, it was revealed that almost two-thirds of questioned patients presented nocebo effect after elimination diet, which seems to have same significant influence on performing DBPC during gluten challenge [29,33].

The fact that numerous symptoms manifested by active NCGS can be either vague or simply mimic other medical conditions, makes the diagnostic process long lasting and complex. For instance, bloating, abdominal pain, and irregular bowel movements are typical symptoms seen in IBS [20]. The overlapping symptoms of IBS, Crohn's disease and GRD are shown in Figure 3.

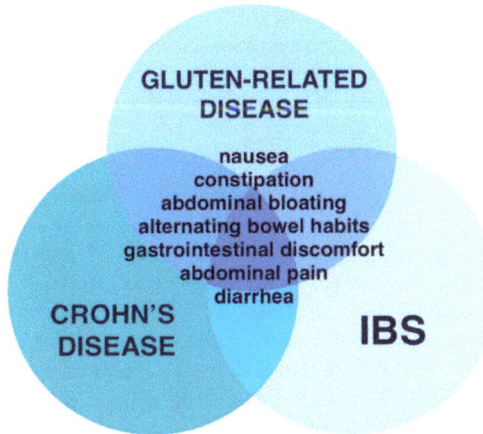

Figure 3. Overlapping symptoms in Crohn's disease, IBS and gluten-related disease.

The similarity between symptomatology of IBS and NCGS may lead to a wrong diagnosis and ineffective treatment [6]. The clinical case described by Vojdani and Perlmutter, presented a 49-year-old woman formerly diagnosed with IBS. The patient complained about abdominal pain, constipation, acid reflux and headache. Following conditions were contemplated and finally excluded: autoimmunological disorders, abnormal level of thyroid hormones, *H. pylori* infection [34]. Consequently, in the course of inappropriate therapy, the patient developed symptoms imitating systemic lupus erythematosus. Furthermore, the patient showed some improvement after corticosteroids administration, which appeared to be confusing for making right diagnosis as well [34]. Ultimately, after years of inappropriate treatment, the NCGS turned out to be the reason for patient's affliction. In addition, a few studies indicate that NCGS can be primary trigger for developing IBS. Virtually, as NCGS and IBS-like symptoms tend to overlap, the diagnostic process is particularly challenging [20,35,36].

Even though the diagnosis within the wide spectrum of bowel diseases was made, in the case of continuous therapy failure, it is crucial to reconsider NCGS as the possible cause. A clinical case of a patient with NCGS overlapping Crohn's disease has been reported. The onset of Crohn's disease is characterized mainly by unspecific symptoms, including diarrhea, weight loss, right lower quadrant abdominal pain, which proceed in a gradual way, with very harmful effects [37]. In the above-mentioned case report, the patient suffered from refractory Crohn's disease for 14 years and elevated IgG class antibodies directed against native gliadin (AGA) were detected, which shed a light on gluten related disorder. Introduction of GFD ceased diarrhea and enabled the patient to gain weight [34]. It is worth highlighting that NCGS patients are twice as likely to have AGA positivity [38].

At present, the linkage between gluten sensitivity, such as CD, and neurological disorders seems to be obvious. So far, numerous studies have unveiled extra intestinal symptoms affecting the peripheral and central nervous system due to celiac sprue. Although not fully understood yet, a wide range of NCGS neurological complications has been reported too. The state-of-the-art knowledge on NCGS revealed its association with transient and subtle cognitive impairment, being called "brain fog" [39]. Some scientists suggest NCGS to worsen symptoms in the context of depression but further examination must be performed to comprehend and determine NCGS relation with depressive disorders [32]. Busby et al. in their meta-analysis pointed out that standardization of methods measuring dietary adherence and mood symptoms is vital in terms of future research. Nevertheless, they admit that the gluten elimination diet may be an applicable treatment for mood disorders in patients suffering from gluten-related diseases [40].

It has not been until recently, when researchers explored that NCGS may be associated with gluten ataxia (GA), as the patients with typical GA symptoms did not meet criteria for CD diagnosis [41]. NCGS symptoms are believed to originate from an innate immune response. Interestingly, autoimmune diseases are reported to be more frequent in this group of patients, comparing to sheer IBS patients [42].

3. Results

Comparison of selected clinical trials concerning NCGS is shown in Table 2. In the study by Capannolo et al. patients with CD and WA were excluded while in the study by Elli et al. patients without CD, WA, IBS were enrolled. The prevalence of NCGS, CD and WA among patients with functional GI symptoms in the study of Capannolo et al. was estimated to be 6.88%, 6.63% and 0.51%. Capannolo et al. indicate that high frequency of visits due to gluten-related symptoms is not associated with high prevalence of GRDs. Ellie et al. established that 14% of patients, suspected to have NCGS because of responding to gluten withdrawal showed a symptomatic relapse during the gluten challenge. It was highlighted that GFD can have a beneficial effect even in the absence of CD or WA. However, there are certain limitations seen in both of compared above research papers. The research of Capannolo et al. was lacking blindness in GFD challenge and missing evaluation of possible influence of other food components. Besides it was conducted before Salerno Criteria were introduced (2015). A choice of timing and gluten dosage shown in the research of Elli et al. was not in line with the timing suggested by Salerno criteria. In addition, the protocol did not make use of a scheduled diet besides GFD. Moreover, a nocebo effect may be presumed, in consistence with symptomatic deterioration observed in the placebo group. Other diet variables in both studies cannot be excluded (ATIs) [43,44].

Table 2. Comparison of selected researches on NCGS.

References	Study Group	Exclusion Criteria	Methods	Findings	Comments
Biesiekierski et al. 2013	IBS patients fulfilling Rome III criteria in NCCS criteria, on GFD for 6 weeks	CD, IBD, age < 16, serious GI disease (cirrhosis), psychiatric disorders, alcohol abuse, NSAIDs and immunosuppressive treatment	GFD for 6 weeks, next 2-weeks diet low in FODMAPs, then 3 days one of the groups—high gluten 16 g, low gluten 2 g gluten or 14 g whey protein, control for 2 weeks washout period and crossover to another group for 3 days. **The primary outcome**: GI symptoms measured by using 100-mm VAS scoring. **The secondary outcome**: Fatigue measured by Daily-Fatigue Impact Scale (D-FIS), gliadin-specific T-cell response, biomarkers.	**The primary outcome**: Gluten-specific responses only in 8% of patients, 16% had worsening of overall GI symptoms in high gluten diet. **The secondary outcome**: Fatigue measured by D-FIS was lower in the low FOTMAPs diet, no significant difference in biomarkers, physical activity or sleep was observed, only one patient had gliadin-specific T-cell response.	**Limitations**: The nocebo effect was present independent of substances which was delivered
Capannolo et al. 2014	Individuals with gluten related symptoms	CD and WA	NCGS finding: on the basis of the disappearance of the symptoms within GFD 6 month, followed by 1month GD.	CD patients: 26 (6.63%); **WA** patients: 2 (0.51%); **NCGS** patients: 27 (6.88%). Patients with **no change of symptoms after GFD** 337 (85.9%) **Symptoms in 74% NCGS patients:** **Intestinal**: abdominal pain, diarrhea, constipation, alternating bowel function, epigastric pain **Extra intestinal**: malaise, chronic fatigue, headache, anxiety, confused mind, depression, joint/muscle pain, resembling fibromyalgia, weight loss, anemia, dermatitis, rash **Related disorders in NCGS patients**: lactose intolerance, autoimmune thyroiditis, type 1 diabetes, psoriasis, sarcoidosis	**Limitations**: Lack of blindness in GFD challenge Missing evaluation of possible influence by other food components
Zanini et al. 2015	Individuals on gluten-free diet (GFD) on their own initiative	CD, non-strict adherence to a GFD, symptomatic on GFD	The primary outcome: the ability of the participants to correctly identify flour containing gluten. GSRS questionnaire was performed	Only 34% (12 participants) correctly identified gluten- containing flour fulfilling the clinical diagnostic criteria for NCCS.	The gluten-free flour used in this test contained FODMAP
Hollon et al. 2015	Individuals with Active CD, CD in Remission, Gluten Sensitivity (GS)	Positive CD serology, abnormal duodenal histopathology, unresponsive to gluten open challenge	GS finding: on the basis of the disappearance of the symptoms within GFD: non-blinded gluten challenge (10 g) for a minimum of 2 months before endoscopy	Increase of gut permeability after PT-gliadin ex-vivo administration in all three study groups, and in control group	**Limitations**: Lack of blindness in GFD challenge—possible placebo-response; Lack of GFD challenge in the control group—possible individuals with undiagnosed GS/CD
Shahbazkhani et al. 2015	Individuals with newly diagnosed IBS based on the Rome III criteria	Patients with CD, GFD introduced ever in medical history, self-exclusion of wheat from the diet, IBD, diabetes, concurrent drugs for depression/anxiety, NSAI drugs intake, abnormal levels of: glucose, urea, creatinine, sodium, potassium, hemoglobin, erythrocyte sedimentation rate, thyroid function tests	GS finding: IBS diagnosed patients responding to gluten challenge by means of statistically significant worsening of symptoms after gluten meal packet. Patients previously following strict GFD, continued gluten challenge for 6 weeks	Significant increase for following symptoms after gluten-containing meal challenge: bloating, abdominal pain, stool consistence, tiredness, nausea	**Limitations**: Packets containing gluten meal in the form of powder—not recommended according to Salerno criteria **Pros**: double-blind randomized placebo-controlled trial

Table 2. Cont.

References	Study Group	Exclusion Criteria	Methods	Findings	Comments
Di Sabatino et al. 2015	Suspected NCGS individuals	CD, WA	Individuals were randomly assigned to groups given gluten or placebo for 1 week, each via gastro-soluble capsules. After a 1 week of gluten-free diet, participants crossed over to the other group.	Gluten group: significantly increased overall symptoms (intestinal symptoms: abdominal bloating and pain, extra-intestinal symptoms: foggy mind, depression, aphthous stomatitis) vs. placebo group.	**Limitation:** small study group
Elli et al. 2016	Individuals with functional gastroenterological symptoms with enrolled on 3-week-long GFD	CD, WA, IBS psychiatric disorders, major abdominal surgery, diabetes mellitus, systemic autoimmune diseases, previous anaphylactic episodes, any systemic disorders, pregnant, breast feeding women, GFD in previous 6 months, patients on pharmacological therapy	Phase 1. GFD response individuals: questionnaire and next 3-week GFD. Patients with significantly improvement carried on to next phase. Phase 2. 98 subjects. GFD response patients—maintain strict GFD and underwent placebo-controlled double-blind gluten challenge with crossover. Patients were randomized to take gluten in capsules or placebo (rice starch) for 7 days. Total duration: 21 days: 7 days on gluten or placebo, 7 days wash-out, 7 days on gluten or placebo.	28 individuals from phase 2 reported a symptomatic relapse and deterioration of quality of life. 14 patients responded to the placebo ingestion. About 14 patients responding to gluten withdrawal showed a symptomatic relapse during the gluten challenge—they are suspected to have NCGS.	**Strengths:** The blinding of patients and doctors, and the crossover design. **Weaknesses:** arbitrary choice of timing and gluten dosage, the protocol did not make use of a scheduled diet besides GFD, other diet variables cannot be excluded (ATIs). Symptomatic deterioration was also observed in placebo group.
Rosinach et al. 2016	Individuals with clinical GI symptoms and clinical and histological remission after GFD	Age < 18, CD, NSAIDs and Olmesartan immunosuppressive treatment in last month, immunosuppressive therapy, parasitic or H. pylori infection, AD, pregnant or breastfeeding women, participation in other randomized controlled trials in the last 4 weeks, serious GI diseases and GI surgery, severe comorbidities, failure to comply with the protocol requirements	Patients were randomly assigned to gluten group (20 g/day, n = 11) and placebo (n = 7). Clinical symptoms were measured by VAS, quality of life using GIQLI. Scientists examined the presence of gamma/delta+ cells and transglutaminase deposits. primary end-point: disease relapse after 6 months	91% of patients with clinical relapse during gluten challenge compared to 28.5% after placebo. Worsening results in clinical scores and GIQLI was observed in patients on gluten diet, but not in the placebo	**Limitations:** a small study group
Carroccio et al. 2017	Individuals with NCWS		Data collecting from a previous study of NCWS.	88% subjects improved after a diagnosis of NCWS; 145 of 148 patients on strict GFD (98%) had reduced symptoms, compared to 30 of 52 patients who were not on GFD, 20 (from 22) subjects who repeated DBPC challenge reacted to wheat. NCWS is a persistent condition.	**Limitations:** not thoroughly discussed exclusion criteria
Skodje et al. 2018	Individuals self-reported NCGS on gluten-free diet (GFD) on their own initiative for at least 6 months	Exclusion criteria: CD, WA, IBD, gastrointestinal comorbidity, alcohol abuse, pregnancy, breast feeding, women in fertile age without contraception, long travel distance, considerable infection, patients on immunosuppressive agents' therapy	GFD for 6 months, next 7 days on one of three diets challenge (gluten 5.7g, fructans 2.1g and placebo), 7 days washout, then crossover to next diet. The primary outcome: gastrointestinal symptoms measured by GSRS-IBS. The secondary outcome: daily GI symptoms measured by VAS, life quality depends on symptoms by SF-36, depression and anxiety symptoms measured by Hospital Anxiety and Depression Scale, Fatigue measured by Giessen Subjective Complaint List and VAS	**The primary outcome:** overall CSRS-IBS higher in the fructans group (38.6) than in the gluten group (33.1) and placebo (34.3). **The secondary outcome:** overall GI symptoms measured by VAS higher in FODMAP's diet, decreased vitality and greater weakness in the group of patients receiving fructans	**Limitations:** high nocebo response

Table 2. *Cont.*

References	Study Group	Exclusion Criteria	Methods	Findings	Comments
Roncoroni et al. 2019	Individuals with NCGS criteria, complaining about functional GI symptoms	CD, WA, IBD, adult age (<18 years old), positive anti-tissue transglutaminase IgA, psychiatric disorders, major abdominal surgery, diabetes, GFD for previous six months, autoimmune diseases and systemic disorders, pregnancy, breast feeding, experience of anaphylaxis and patients during pharmacotherapy	GFD for 3 weeks, then exposure to diets with gradually increasing the amount of gluten: low-gluten diet (3.5–4 g gluten/day, week 1, n = 22 + 2 dropped out patients), mid-gluten diet (6.7–8 g gluten/day, week 2, n = 14), and a high-gluten diet (10–13 g gluten/day, week 3, n = 8). Patients without GI symptoms on a previous diet were classified into more gluten-containing diet. Patients with GI symptoms were shifted back to a well-tolerated diet. Daily GI symptoms measured by VAS, life quality depends on symptoms by SF-36	Different reactions of patients after the introduction of gluten.	Limitation: a small study group

In 2015, Zanini et al. published a prospective, randomized, double-blind, placebo-controlled study on patients without CD or wheat allergy as seen in Table 2. Scientists observed 35 patients (31 females and 4 males) being on a GFD due to their own initiative because of gastrointestinal symptoms they had had on a diet containing gluten. They were switched to a diet containing gluten. Participants' ability to distinguish between flours containing gluten and gluten-free was assessed, as well as their score in the Gastrointestinal Symptoms Rating Scale (GSRS). In order to participate in the study, patients had to be over 6 months a self-prescribed GFD and have a Gastrointestinal Symptoms Rating Scale (GSRS) below 4. The CD had had to be excluded before the start of the GFD. Before the beginning of the study t-TG antibody levels were measured and patients were instructed how to keep a diet diary. After 3 months, t-TG antibody level was checked again and GSRS questionnaire was performed. The participants received 10-g sachets containing gluten-free or gluten- containing flour labeled A or B. Patients were ordered to add contents to the pasta or soup for 10 days. Then for 2 weeks there was a washout period. Then, the patients received a second sachet with the other label, which they were to consume for 10 days. The primary outcome was the ability of the participants to correctly identify flour containing gluten. The study showed that only 34% (12 participants) correctly identified gluten- containing flour. Two thirds of the participants were not able to properly identify flour containing gluten. Almost half of the participants 17 (49%) misidentified gluten-free flour as gluten-containing flour, but those patients recorded symptoms and their GSRS scores increased on the flour not containing gluten. The gluten-free flour used in this test contained FODMAP [45].

Hollon et al. in their study (Table 2) disclosure ex-vivo gliadin effect on gut permeability in patients with active celiac disease (ACD), remission celiac disease (RCD) and gluten sensitivity (GS). The results of the research indicated that in all four groups, including control group (NG), there is certain response to gluten administration [46]. Researchers reported increased permeability particularly comparing ACD and GS groups to RCD, which is due to gluten induced alteration of intestinal barrier. Furthermore, researchers by means of quantification method investigated changes in following cytokines IL-6, IL-8, IFN-γ, TNF-α, which showed no significant difference, however, in this case a short period of incubation could implicate results. It should be emphasized that lack of blindness in GFD challenge while recruiting GS group along with lack of GFD challenge in the control group are important limitation in discussed study and could impact final results [46].

Shahbazkhani et al. investigated the relationship between dietary habits in IBS patients and consequent symptom fluctuations (Table 2). In particular researchers were interested in gluten impact on wellbeing of IBS patients and weather it may induce IBS-like symptoms. After rigid inclusion and exclusion criteria, strict six-week GFD 72 patients were recruited and divided into two groups: gluten containing group (study group), gluten free group (placebo group). Symptoms were analyzed by means of visual analogue scale (VAS). The results of the research revealed significant worsening of symptoms in a study group after gluten powder challenge. Scientists reported increase of overall symptoms such as satisfaction with stool consistency, tiredness, nausea, bloating in study group comparing to the control one. The results occurred to be statistically significant [47]. Nevertheless, there was limitation such as gluten form—a packet of 100 g powder, which is not recommended anymore by Salerno criteria [29].

According to the study published in Gastroenterology, scientists discovered that FODMAPs are another wheat antigen along with gluten triggering symptoms in patients with NCGS. Biesiekierski et al. conducted a double-blind crossover trial in which participated 37 patients suffering from NCGS and IBD. The following exclusion criteria were applied: age less than 16 years, CD confirmed by genetic tests and duodenal biopsy, alcohol abuse, chronic non-steroidal anti-inflammatory drugs (NSAIDs) and immunosuppressant treatment, uncontrolled psychiatric illness. Patients who had confirmed symptoms of IBS by accomplished the Rome III criteria and symptoms well controlled on a GFD were qualified for the study. Another requirement was to follow the GFD 6 weeks before this clinical trial. The first stage of the study was identical for all participants and the task was consuming for a one week a gluten-free and low FODMAPs diet. After a 2-week washout period, patients were randomly assigned to the three groups: high-gluten, low-gluten and placebo, without introducing FODMAP into the diet. The symptoms of the patients were measured by using 100-mm VAS scoring and Daily-Fatigue Impact Scale (D-FIS). All participants were asked to return to the second stage of this study—trial in which all patients received each diets for 3-days [48]. Gluten-specific responses were found only in 8% of patients. Scientists found a high nocebo effect and reproducibility of induction of symptoms in each arm was low [48].

Biesiekierski et al. noticed that patients with NCGS do not present a statistically significant occurrence of symptoms after introducing gluten into the diet, if at the same time they limit products rich in FODMAP (Table 2). These results may suggest that the symptoms in patients suffering from NCGS may in many cases be associated with intolerance to the contained sugars, but not hypersensitivity to gluten. Surprisingly, the patients involved into study evinced eminently high VAS ratings for their symptoms, despite being on GFD. Furthermore, an anticipatory nocebo response could influence the final results of this DBPC research. It is interesting that all participants eventually returned to GFD at the end of the trail as they 'subjectively describe feeling better' [48].

Scientists from Oslo, Skodje et al., conducted a study in which took part 59 patients on a GFD, in whom CD was excluded (Table 2). Participants were divided into three groups: receiving diet including gluten (5.7 g), fructans (2.1 g) and placebo. The clinical trial lasted 7 days and was preceded by a 1-week washout period. The following symptoms were recorded: pain, bloating, diarrhea, constipation, nausea, dizziness, weakness, sleepiness and tiredness. Participants filled a questionnaire containing 13 questions about their gastrointestinal symptoms and filled VAS. The results were measured by GSRS, Irritable Bowel Syndrome scale (GSRS-IBS), VAS, Short Form-36 (SF-36) and Giessen Subjective Complaint List [49]. Scientists observed that daily symptoms calculated using VAS score were significantly higher in fructans diet. Furthermore, they noticed that overall GSRS-IBS was higher in the FODMAPs group (38.6 g) than in the gluten group (33.1 g) and placebo (34.3 g). More ailments were recorded in the group receiving fructans, compered to two another groups. In addition, it was demonstrated that a diet rich in FODMAPSs caused greater weakness and decreased vitality compared to the placebo and gluten groups. The results of the study indicate that FODMAPs are a trigger factor of gastrointestinal complaints in patients suffering from NCGS [49]. Thus, scientists are leaning towards renaming NCGS to a more recent NCWS [27].

Di Sabatino et al. observed increased severity of intestinal symptoms (abdominal bloating, abdominal pain) and extra intestinal symptoms (foggy mind, depression, and aphthous stomatitis) among subjects with suspected NCGS (excluded CD and WA). Although, this study did not make a significant contribution in development of knowledge about NCGS and had some weaknesses such as lack of a control group, it indicates possible symptoms experienced by NCGS patients (Table 2) [50].

In order to prove that gluten is a trigger factor in patients with NCGS, Rosinach et al. conducted a study in which 18 participants were assigned to gluten or placebo groups. In 10 out of 11 patients, symptoms worsened in response to a gluten-containing diet, 7 of which were withdrawn from the study due to the severity of the symptoms [51]. There was no early termination in the placebo group although in 2 participants symptoms were observed (Table 2) [51].

Carroccio et al. collected and analyzed data from 200 patients examined in previous study with diagnosed NCWS. Their findings are interesting because about 90% of patients who maintained wheat-free diet (WFD) were characterized by significant improvement of IBS symptoms [52]. The authors came to the conclusion that NCWS is a persistent condition and patients with NCWS should therefore be correctly identified and treated with WFD (Table 2) [52].

Roncoroni et al. conducted a study on dietary exposure to different amounts of gluten in patients meeting the criteria of the NCGS [53]. Researchers observed different reactions of patients after the introduction of gluten. Some of them had a worsening of well-being and increased symptoms after a small dose of gluten, others observed this effect after the medium dose and others only after a high dose of gluten (Table 2) [53].

Carrocio et al. in their study in 2011 emphasize the link between particular food ingestion and deteriorating symptoms in a subgroup of IBS patients [54]. It clearly shows alleviation of the symptoms in 22% of IBS patients—whose previous treatment was ineffective—after eliminating gluten from the diet. Moreover, researchers excluded association of DQ2 and DQ8 haplotypes with frequent gluten sensitivity, however, patients presenting food hypersensitivity (FH) to both wheat- and cow's milk-protein were reported to be often DQ2/DQ8 positive. Fecal eosinophil cationic protein (ECP) may be useful while identifying FH in IBS-patients (Table 3) [54].

Carroccio et al. in their study published in 2012 examined individuals with non-celiac WS, diagnosed by DBPC challenge with IBS-like symptoms, compared to CD patients and IBS patients [55]. Authors described presence of two types of WS subjects: WS similar to CD and WS associated with multiple food hypersensitivity. Besides, symptoms such as anemia, weight loss, self-reported wheat intolerance, coexistent atopy, and food allergy in infancy were noticed more often in WS compared to IBS controls. Furthermore, WS individuals were characterized by higher frequency of presence IgG/IgA anti-gliadin in serum, basophil activation (assessed by flow cytometric method) and histology specific eosinophil infiltration of the duodenal and colon mucosa. This study shows the differences between non-celiac WS and other gluten-related disorders (Table 3) [55].

Volta et al. in their study, assessed the level of immunoglobulin distinctive for CD in patients with GS comparing to CD [56]. They revealed that 50% of GS patients presented IgG AGA, whereas IgA AGA was seen only in a few patients in study group. Besides, researchers observed absence of IgA EmA, IgA tTGA, IgG DGP-AGA, which are typical for CD, within GS group (Table 3) [56].

Basing on a study group conducted by Volta et al., Caio et al. continued research on AGA IgG [38]. Scientists aimed to explore GFD impact on AGA IgG titer in AGA IgG positive patients (44 individuals) with NCGS. After six months of GFD AGA IgG disappeared in all the patients (Table 3).

Carrocio et al., in another research conducted in 2015, evaluated and described frequent ANA positivity within NCWS patients group [57]. The study demonstrated ANA positivity occurring along with DQ2/DQ8 haplotypes. As it was previously discussed, DQ2/DQ8 positivity is a distinctive feature of CD rather than NCWS. Thus, researchers highlight the need of intraepithelial intestinal flow cytometric pattern, which is an accurate method identifying seronegative CD patients, in the initial diagnostic biopsy. However, scientists found autoimmune diseases (AD) particularly frequent in study group. Autoimmune thyroiditis was reported to be the most frequent AD and amounted for 22% and 24% in retrospective and prospective groups respectively Table 3) [57].

Infantino et al. similarly to Volta observed frequent IgG AGA occurrence in NCGS patients, however, the author highlights that it is still lacking diagnostic accuracy. Nevertheless, in some cases, it can be helpful in the diagnostic process of NCGS patients [58].

Papers included in Table 3. Indicate IgG AGA and ECP to be helpful diagnostic tool while diagnosing NCGS. Still they have limited application in a large group of NCGS patients and cannot be widely used in NCGS diagnostic protocol [54,58].

Table 3. Researches on potential NCGS biomarkers.

References	Study Group	Exclusion Criteria	Methods	Findings	Comments
Carroccio et al. 2011	Individuals who fulfilled Rome II criteria for IBS	Individuals with organic diseases	Symptom severity questionnaire was analyzed, fecal samples were assayed, and levels of specific immunoglobulin E were measured. Patients were observed for 4 weeks, placed on an elimination diet (without cow's milk and derivatives, wheat, egg, tomato, and chocolate) for 4 weeks, and kept a diet diary. Those who reported improvements after the elimination diet period were then diagnosed with food hypersensitivity (FH), based on the results of a double-blind, placebo-controlled, oral food challenge (with cow's milk proteins and then with wheat proteins).	40 of patients with IBS (25%) were found to have FH. Levels of fecal ECP and tryptase were significantly higher among patients with IBS and FH than those without FH. The ECP assay was the most accurate assay for diagnosis of FH, showing 65% sensitivity and 91% specificity.	Limitations: recruitment of patients not in line with Salerno criteria.
Carroccio et al. 2012	Individuals with non-celiac wheat sensitivity (NCWS),	IgA deficiency, self-exclusion of wheat from the diet, lack of DBPC-challenge method in the diagnosis	A review of the clinical charts of patients with IBS-like presentation, diagnosed with WS challenge in the years 2001-2011.	1/3 IBS patients who underwent DBPC wheat challenge were really suffering from WS. WS group: higher frequency of anemia, weight loss, self-reported wheat intolerance, coexistent atopy, and food allergy in infancy than the IBS controls, higher frequency of positive serum assays for IgG/IgA anti-gliadin and cytometric basophil activation in "in vitro" assay, eosinophil infiltration of the duodenal and colon mucosa. Two groups with distinct clinical characteristics were identified: WS alone (with similar to CD clinical features) and WS with multiple food hypersensitivity (clinical features similar to those found in allergic patients)	Limitations: recruitment of patients not in line with Salerno criteria.
Volta et al. 2012	Individuals with GS (NCGS)	CD, WA	Retrospective evaluation of collected samples from GS (study group) and CD (control group) individuals. Assessment of IgG/IgA AGA, IgA EmA, IgA tTGA, IgG DGP-AGA. HLA DQ2/DQ8 presence was assessed	GS is characterized by IgG AGA positivity (50%), although is less common comparing to CD. IgA AGA are rare. GS patients were lacking EmA, tTGA, and DGP-AGA.	Limitations: not thoroughly described exclusion criteria for study group

Table 3. *Cont.*

References	Study Group	Exclusion Criteria	Methods	Findings	Comments
Caio et al. 2014	Individuals with NCGS with simultaneous AGA IgG positivity	CD, WA	AGA of both IgG and IgA classes were assayed by ELISA in 44 NCGS and 40 CD patients after 6 months of gluten-free diet.	AGA IgG in NCGS patients disappear after introduction of GFD.	
Carroccio et al. 2015	NCWS patients of the retrospective cohort study	Incomplete clinical charts were excluded from retrospective study; for both studies: EmA in the culture medium of the duodenal biopsies, self-exclusion of wheat from the diet and refusal to reintroduce it before entering the study, other organic gastrointestinal diseases.	NCWS patients—tTG IgG, EmA IgA and IgG negative, absence of intestinal villous atrophy and WA. Patient medical records were reviewed to identify those with autoimmune disease (AD). CD or IBS served as controls. Serum samples were collected from all subjects and ANA levels were measured by immunofluorescence analysis. Participants completed a questionnaire and their medical records were reviewed to identify those with ADs. Individuals were randomly assigned to groups given gluten or placebo for 1 week, each via gastro-soluble capsules. After a 1	Patients with NCWS were more likely to be ANA positive than both patients with CD and IBS, in both the retrospective and prospective studies. Patients with NCWS showed a frequency of AD similar to CD, but significantly higher than IBS controls, in both the retrospective and prospective studies. NCWS or CD are more likely to be ANA-positive, have DQ2/DQ8 haplotypes and AD compared with patients with IBS.	Limitations: selection bias of the tertiary centers conducting research; evaluation of the duodenal histology; not in line with Salerno criteria
	NCWS patients of the prospective study				
Infantino et al. 2015	Individuals with suspected NCGS	CD, WA	Evaluation of gluten-free diet in 38 NCGS (study group), 42 CD and 54 HCW (control group) individuals. Assessment of IgG/IgA AGA, IgA EmA, IgA tTGA, IgG/IgA DGP-AGA. HLA DQ2/DQ8 presence was assessed	Statistically significant correlation between AGA IgG and NCGS were found. However, AGA IgG still remains to be weak NCGS marker.	Limitations: recruitment of patients not in line with Salerno criteria; small study group

4. Discussion

Nowadays, a gluten-free diet is fashionable and is promoted by many celebrities. Many people undergo this fashion and despite lack of symptoms, try to reject gluten because they believe it may harm their health. In 2016, as much as USD 15.5 billion was spent on gluten-free food sales. This value is more than twice as high as in 2011. Lack of gluten in food consumed by people who tolerate it well may not bring favorable results.

In a study conducted by Norsa et al., children with CD were tested for at least one year on a GFD diet. As many as 34.8% of children on GFD diet had high concentrations of triglycerides on fasting, 24.1% high concentration of LDL cholesterol and 29.4% increased blood pressure. In 52 out of 114 participants there were available cards with information on blood lipids concentration before GFD introduction. 24% of children on GFD had had LDL cholesterol borderline values. That was much more than before the introduction of the diet (10%). However, these data did not meet the value of statistical significance ($p = 0.09$) [59].

Studies show that gluten may have a positive effect on triglyceride levels. In a clinical trial in which 20 adults with hyperlipidemia took part, a group with a balanced diet and a group with a high gluten content (78 g per day with an average human intake of 10–15 g) were studied. The high gluten diet group had a decreased triglyceride concentration of 19.2% ($p = 0.0003$) compared to the control group after one month of the study [60]. In another study, a group of patients consuming 60 g of gluten per day had a 13% ($p = 0.05$) lower triglyceride concentration compared to the control group [61]. In a study published in 2017, the estimated gluten consumption lead to the protective effect against cardiovascular disease (HR 0.85, 95% CI 0.77-0.93, $p = 0.002$) [62].

Gluten-free products can also be more than twice as expensive as regular products [63]. There are other disadvantages of GFD. The GFD turned out to be poor in trace elements and vitamins, such as zinc, iron, magnesium, calcium, vitamin D, vitamin B_{12}, folate, and fiber [64,65]. Furthermore, Tovoli et al. compared scores obtained by NCWS and CD individuals using quality of life questionnaire (CDQ) before GFD introduction and after at least one year. NCWS patients still reported intestinal and parenteral symptoms, although symptoms were significantly reduced in comparison to period before GFD. Therefore, other factors influencing NCWS should be investigated [66].

Finally, based on revised research results, it is clear that NCGS still remains to be the subject of uncertainty, especially in terms of other wheat components contribution to its symptoms. There are only a few published forms of research in the last six years. It should be stressed that it is hard to compare the results of each study as obtained methods and criteria significantly vary. Moreover, the timing of onset of each research was of a great importance as some of them were conducted before Salerno criteria were introduced, which led to many interpretations and qualification protocols of patients with NCGS-like symptoms. Further investigations and seeking for biomarkers would play key role in improving of the diagnostic process and patients' follow up.

5. Conclusions

1. Symptoms of non-celiac gluten sensitivity are similar to gluten-related disease, irritable bowel syndrome and Crohn's disease.
2. With Salerno Experts' Criteria of non-celiac gluten sensitivity it is possible to diagnose patients properly and give them advice about nutritional treatment.

Author Contributions: Conceptualization, A.R., M.P., B.N.-I.; Methodology and resources A.M., K.B., B.N.-I.; Visualization A.M., M.P., A.R., K.B.; Writing—Review & Editing A.R., M.P., A.M., K.B., B.N.-I.; Software K.B.; Supervision—B.N.-I.

Funding: This research received no external funding.

Conflicts of Interest: The authors declare no conflict of interest.

References

1. Sapone, A.; Bai, J.C.; Ciacci, C.; Dolinsek, J.; Green, P.H.R.; Hadjivassiliou, M.; Kaukinen, K.; Rostami, K.; Sanders, D.S.; Schumann, M.; et al. Spectrum of gluten-related disorders: Consensus on new nomenclature and classification. *BMC Med.* **2012**, *10*, 13. [CrossRef] [PubMed]
2. Alvey, C.; Anderson, C.M.; Freeman, M. Wheat Gluten and Coeliac Disease. *Arch. Dis Child.* **1957**, *32*, 434–437. [CrossRef] [PubMed]
3. Jones, A.L. The Gluten-Free Diet: Fad or Necessity? *Diabetes Spectr. Publ. Am. Diabetes Assoc.* **2017**, *30*, 118–123. [CrossRef] [PubMed]
4. Balakireva, A.V.; Zamyatnin, A.A. Properties of Gluten Intolerance: Gluten Structure, Evolution, Pathogenicity and Detoxification Capabilities. *Nutrients* **2016**, *8*. Available online: https://www.ncbi.nlm.nih.gov/pmc/articles/PMC5084031/ (accessed on 28 January 2019). [CrossRef] [PubMed]
5. Ortiz, C.; Valenzuela, R.; Lucero, A.Y. Celiac disease, non celiac gluten sensitivity and wheat allergy: Comparison of 3 different diseases triggered by the same food. *Rev. Chil. Pediatría* **2017**, *88*, 417–423. [CrossRef] [PubMed]
6. Barbaro, M.R.; Cremon, C.; Stanghellini, V.; Barbara, G. Recent advances in understanding non-celiac gluten sensitivity. *F1000Research* **2018**, *7*. [CrossRef] [PubMed]
7. Catassi, C.; Bai, J.C.; Bonaz, B.; Bouma, G.; Calabrò, A.; Carroccio, A.; Castillejo, G.; Ciacci, C.; Cristofori, F.; Dolinsek, J.; et al. Non-Celiac Gluten Sensitivity: The New Frontier of Gluten Related Disorders. *Nutrients* **2013**, *5*, 3839–3853. [CrossRef] [PubMed]
8. Cooper, B.T.; Holmes, G.K.; Ferguson, R.; Thompson, R.A.; Allan, R.N.; Cooke, W.T. Gluten-sensitive diarrhea without evidence of celiac disease. *Gastroenterology* **1980**, *79*, 801–806. [CrossRef]
9. Ludvigsson, J.F.; Leffler, D.A.; Bai, J.; Biagi, F.; Fasano, A.; Green, P.H.; Hadjivassiliou, M.; Kaukinen, K.; Kelly, C.P.; Leonard, J.N.; et al. The Oslo definitions for coeliac disease and related terms. *Gut* **2013**, *62*, 43–52. [CrossRef]
10. Ierardi, E.; Losurdo, G.; Piscitelli, D.; Giorgio, F.; Amoruso, A.; Iannone, A.; Principi, M.; Di Leo, A. Biological markers for non-celiac gluten sensitivity: A question awaiting for a convincing answer. *Gastroenterol. Hepatol. Bed Bench.* **2018**, *11*, 203–208.
11. Leccioli, V.; Oliveri, M.; Romeo, M.; Berretta, M.; Rossi, P. A New Proposal for the Pathogenic Mechanism of Non-Coeliac/Non-Allergic Gluten/Wheat Sensitivity: Piecing Together the Puzzle of Recent Scientific Evidence. *Nutrients* **2019**, *9*. Available online: https://www.ncbi.nlm.nih.gov/pmc/articles/PMC5707675/ (accessed on 28 January 2019). [CrossRef] [PubMed]
12. Tanveer, M.; Ahmed, A. Non-Celiac Gluten Sensitivity: A Systematic Review. *J. Coll Physicians Surg.–Pak. Jcpsp* **2019**, *29*, 51–57. [CrossRef] [PubMed]
13. Singh, P.; Arora, A.; Strand, T.A.; Leffler, D.A.; Catassi, C.; Green, P.H.; Kelly, C.P.; Ahuja, V.; Makharia, G.K. Global Prevalence of Celiac Disease: Systematic Review and Meta-analysis. *Clin. Gastroenterol. Hepatol. Off. Clin. Pr. J. Am. Gastroenterol. Assoc.* **2018**, *16*, 823–836.e2. [CrossRef] [PubMed]
14. Elli, L.; Branchi, F.; Tomba, C.; Villalta, D.; Norsa, L.; Ferretti, F.; Roncoroni, L.; Bardella, M.T. Diagnosis of gluten related disorders: Celiac disease, wheat allergy and non-celiac gluten sensitivity. *World J. Gastroenterol.* **2015**, *21*, 7110–7119. [CrossRef] [PubMed]
15. Carroccio, A.; Giambalvo, O.; La Blasca, F.; Iacobucci, R.; D'Alcamo, A.; Mansueto, P. Self-Reported Non-Celiac Wheat Sensitivity in High School Students: Demographic and Clinical Characteristics. *Nutrients* **2017**, *9*. Available online: https://www.ncbi.nlm.nih.gov/pmc/articles/PMC5537885/ (accessed on 28 January 2019). [CrossRef] [PubMed]
16. Cabrera-Chávez, F.; Dezar, G.V.A.; Islas-Zamorano, A.P.; Espinoza-Alderete, J.G.; Vergara-Jiménez, M.J.; Magaña-Ordorica, D.; Ontiveros, N. Prevalence of Self-Reported Gluten Sensitivity and Adherence to a Gluten-Free Diet in Argentinian Adult Population. *Nutrients* **2017**, *9*, 81. [CrossRef] [PubMed]
17. DiGiacomo, D.V.; Tennyson, C.A.; Green, P.H.; Demmer, R.T. Prevalence of gluten-free diet adherence among individuals without celiac disease in the USA: Results from the Continuous National Health and Nutrition Examination Survey 2009–2010. *Scand. J. Gastroenterol.* **2013**, *48*, 921–925. [CrossRef] [PubMed]
18. Van Gils, T.; Nijeboer, P.; IJssennagger, C.E.; Sanders, D.S.; Mulder, C.J.J.; Bouma, G. Prevalence and Characterization of Self-Reported Gluten Sensitivity in The Netherlands. *Nutrients* **2016**, *8*. Available online: https://www.ncbi.nlm.nih.gov/pmc/articles/PMC5133100/ (accessed on 28 January 2019). [CrossRef]

19. Aziz, I.; Lewis, N.R.; Hadjivassiliou, M.; Winfield, S.N.; Rugg, N.; Kelsall, A.; Newrick, L.; Sanders, D.S. A UK study assessing the population prevalence of self-reported gluten sensitivity and referral characteristics to secondary care. *Eur J. Gastroenterol. Hepatol.* **2014**, *26*, 33–39. [CrossRef]
20. Volta, U.; Bardella, M.T.; Calabrò, A.; Troncone, R.; Corazza, G.R.; Study Group for Non-Celiac Gluten Sensitivity. An Italian prospective multicenter survey on patients suspected of having non-celiac gluten sensitivity. *BMC Med.* **2014**, *12*, 85. [CrossRef]
21. Reese, I.; Schäfer, C.; Kleine-Tebbe, J.; Ahrens, B.; Bachmann, O.; Ballmer-Weber, B.; Beyer, K.; Bischoff, S.C.; Blümchen, K.; Dölle, S.; et al. Non-celiac gluten/wheat sensitivity (NCGS)-a currently undefined disorder without validated diagnostic criteria and of unknown prevalence: Position statement of the task force on food allergy of the German Society of Allergology and Clinical Immunology (DGAKI). *Allergo J. Int.* **2018**, *27*, 147–151. [PubMed]
22. Biesiekierski, J.R. What is gluten? *J. Gastroenterol. Hepatol.* **2017**, *32* (Suppl 1), 78–81. [CrossRef] [PubMed]
23. Junker, Y.; Zeissig, S.; Kim, S.-J.; Barisani, D.; Wieser, H.; Leffler, D.A.; Zevallos, V.; Libermann, T.A.; Dillon, S.; Freitag, T.L.; et al. Wheat amylase trypsin inhibitors drive intestinal inflammation via activation of toll-like receptor 4. *J. Exp. Med.* **2012**, *209*, 2395–2408. [CrossRef] [PubMed]
24. Barrett, J.S. Extending our knowledge of fermentable, short-chain carbohydrates for managing gastrointestinal symptoms. *Nutr. Clin. Pr. Off. Publ. Am. Soc. Parenter. Enter. Nutr.* **2013**, *28*, 300–306. [CrossRef] [PubMed]
25. Dieterich, W.; Schuppan, D.; Schink, M.; Schwappacher, R.; Wirtz, S.; Agaimy, A.; Neurath, M.F.; Zopf, Y. Influence of low FODMAP and gluten-free diets on disease activity and intestinal microbiota in patients with non-celiac gluten sensitivity. *Clin. Nutr. Edinb Scotl.* **2019**, *38*, 697–707. [CrossRef] [PubMed]
26. Gearry, R.B.; Irving, P.M.; Barrett, J.S.; Nathan, D.M.; Shepherd, S.J.; Gibson, P.R. Reduction of dietary poorly absorbed short-chain carbohydrates (FODMAPs) improves abdominal symptoms in patients with inflammatory bowel disease-a pilot study. *J. Crohns Colitis* **2009**, *3*, 8–14. [CrossRef] [PubMed]
27. Priyanka, P.; Gayam, S.; Kupec, J.T. The Role of a Low Fermentable Oligosaccharides, Disaccharides, Monosaccharides, and Polyol Diet in Nonceliac Gluten Sensitivity. *Gastroenterol. Res. Pract.* **2018**, *2018*, 1561476. [CrossRef] [PubMed]
28. Catassi, G.; Lionetti, E.; Gatti, S.; Catassi, C. The Low FODMAP Diet: Many Question Marks for a Catchy Acronym. *Nutrients* **2017**, *9*, 292. [CrossRef] [PubMed]
29. Catassi, C.; Elli, L.; Bonaz, B.; Bouma, G.; Carroccio, A.; Castillejo, G.; Cellier, C.; Cristofori, F.; de Magistris, L.; Dolinsek, J.; et al. Diagnosis of Non-Celiac Gluten Sensitivity (NCGS): The Salerno Experts' Criteria. *Nutrients* **2015**, *7*, 4966–4977. [CrossRef]
30. Guandalini, S.; Polanco, I. Nonceliac gluten sensitivity or wheat intolerance syndrome? *J. Pediatr.* **2015**, *166*, 805–811. [CrossRef]
31. Volta, U.; Caio, G.; De Giorgio, R.; Henriksen, C.; Skodje, G.; Lundin, K.E. Non-celiac gluten sensitivity: A work-in-progress entity in the spectrum of wheat-related disorders. *Best Pr. Res. Clin. Gastroenterol.* **2015**, *29*, 477–491. [CrossRef] [PubMed]
32. Slim, M.; Rico-Villademoros, F.; Calandre, E.P. Psychiatric Comorbidity in Children and Adults with Gluten-Related Disorders: A Narrative Review. *Nutrients* **2018**, *10*, 875. [CrossRef] [PubMed]
33. Carroccio, A.; Brusca, I.; Mansueto, P.; Pirrone, G.; Barrale, M.; Di Prima, L.; Ambrosiano, G.; Iacono, G.; Lospalluti, M.L.; La Chiusa, S.M.; et al. A cytologic assay for diagnosis of food hypersensitivity in patients with irritable bowel syndrome. *Clin. Gastroenterol. Hepatol. Off. Clin. Pr. J. Am. Gastroenterol. Assoc.* **2010**, *8*, 254–260. [CrossRef]
34. Vojdani, A.; Perlmutter, D. Differentiation between Celiac Disease, Nonceliac Gluten Sensitivity, and Their Overlapping with Crohn's Disease: A Case Series. *Case Rep. Immunol.* **2013**, *2013*, 248482. [CrossRef] [PubMed]
35. Makharia, A.; Catassi, C.; Makharia, G.K. The Overlap between Irritable Bowel Syndrome and Non-Celiac Gluten Sensitivity: A Clinical Dilemma. *Nutrients* **2015**, *7*, 10417–10426. [CrossRef] [PubMed]
36. Catassi, C.; Alaedini, A.; Bojarski, C.; Bonaz, B.; Bouma, G.; Carroccio, A.; Castillejo, G.; De Magistris, L.; Dieterich, W.; Di Liberto, D.; et al. The Overlapping Area of Non-Celiac Gluten Sensitivity (NCGS) and Wheat-Sensitive Irritable Bowel Syndrome (IBS): An Update. *Nutrients* **2017**, *9*. Available online: https://www.ncbi.nlm.nih.gov/pmc/articles/PMC5707740/ (accessed on 27 January 2019). [CrossRef] [PubMed]
37. Torres, J.; Mehandru, S.; Colombel, J.-F.; Peyrin-Biroulet, L. Crohn's disease. *Lancet* **2017**, *389*, 1741–1755. [CrossRef]

38. Caio, G.; Volta, U.; Tovoli, F.; De Giorgio, R. Effect of gluten free diet on immune response to gliadin in patients with non-celiac gluten sensitivity. *BMC Gastroenterol.* **2014**, *14*, 26. [CrossRef]
39. Makhlouf, S.; Messelmani, M.; Zaouali, J.; Mrissa, R. Cognitive impairment in celiac disease and non-celiac gluten sensitivity: Review of literature on the main cognitive impairments, the imaging and the effect of gluten free diet. *Acta Neurol. Belg.* **2018**, *118*, 21–27. [CrossRef]
40. Busby, E.; Bold, J.; Fellows, L.; Rostami, K. Mood Disorders and Gluten: It's Not All in Your Mind! A Systematic Review with Meta-Analysis. *Nutrients* **2018**, *10*, 1708. [CrossRef]
41. Rodrigo, L.; Hernández-Lahoz, C.; Lauret, E.; Rodriguez-Peláez, M.; Soucek, M.; Ciccocioppo, R.; Kruzliak, P. Gluten ataxia is better classified as non-celiac gluten sensitivity than as celiac disease: A comparative clinical study. *Immunol. Res.* **2016**, *64*, 558–564. [CrossRef] [PubMed]
42. Hadjivassiliou, M.; Rao, D.G.; Grìnewald, R.A.; Aeschlimann, D.P.; Sarrigiannis, P.G.; Hoggard, N.; Aeschlimann, P.; Mooney, P.D.; Sanders, D.S. Neurological Dysfunction in Coeliac Disease and Non-Coeliac Gluten Sensitivity. *Am. J. Gastroenterol.* **2016**, *111*, 561–567. [CrossRef] [PubMed]
43. Capannolo, A.; Viscido, A.; Barkad, M.A.; Valerii, G.; Ciccone, F.; Melideo, D.; Frieri, G.; Latella, G. Non-Celiac Gluten Sensitivity among Patients Perceiving Gluten-Related Symptoms. *Digestion* **2015**, *92*, 8–13. [CrossRef] [PubMed]
44. Elli, L.; Tomba, C.; Branchi, F.; Roncoroni, L.; Lombardo, V.; Bardella, M.T.; Ferretti, F.; Conte, D.; Valiante, F.; Fini, L.; et al. Evidence for the Presence of Non-Celiac Gluten Sensitivity in Patients with Functional Gastrointestinal Symptoms: Results from a Multicenter Randomized Double-Blind Placebo-Controlled Gluten Challenge. *Nutrients* **2016**, *8*, 84. [CrossRef] [PubMed]
45. Zanini, B.; Baschè, R.; Ferraresi, A.; Ricci, C.; Lanzarotto, F.; Marullo, M.; Villanacci, V.; Hidalgo, A.; Lanzini, A. Randomised clinical study: Gluten challenge induces symptom recurrence in only a minority of patients who meet clinical criteria for non-coeliac gluten sensitivity. *Aliment. Pharm. Ther.* **2015**, *42*, 968–976. [CrossRef]
46. Hollon, J.; Puppa, E.L.; Greenwald, B.; Goldberg, E.; Guerrerio, A.; Fasano, A. Effect of gliadin on permeability of intestinal biopsy explants from celiac disease patients and patients with non-celiac gluten sensitivity. *Nutrients* **2015**, *7*, 1565–1576. [CrossRef] [PubMed]
47. Shahbazkhani, B.; Sadeghi, A.; Malekzadeh, R.; Khatavi, F.; Etemadi, M.; Kalantri, E.; Rostami-Nejad, M.; Rostami, K. Non-Celiac Gluten Sensitivity Has Narrowed the Spectrum of Irritable Bowel Syndrome: A Double-Blind Randomized Placebo-Controlled Trial. *Nutrients* **2015**, *7*, 4542–4554. [CrossRef]
48. Biesiekierski, J.R.; Peters, S.L.; Newnham, E.D.; Rosella, O.; Muir, J.G.; Gibson, P.R. No effects of gluten in patients with self-reported non-celiac gluten sensitivity after dietary reduction of fermentable, poorly absorbed, short-chain carbohydrates. *Gastroenterology* **2013**, *145*, 320–328.e1-3. [CrossRef]
49. Skodje, G.I.; Sarna, V.K.; Minelle, I.H.; Rolfsen, K.L.; Muir, J.G.; Gibson, P.R.; Veierød, M.B.; Henriksen, C.; Lundin, K.E.A. Fructan, Rather Than Gluten, Induces Symptoms in Patients with Self-Reported Non-Celiac Gluten Sensitivity. *Gastroenterology* **2018**, *154*, 529–539.e2. [CrossRef]
50. Di Sabatino, A.; Volta, U.; Salvatore, C.; Biancheri, P.; Caio, G.; De Giorgio, R.; Di Stefano, M.; Corazza, G.R. Small Amounts of Gluten in Subjects with Suspected Nonceliac Gluten Sensitivity: A Randomized, Double-Blind, Placebo-Controlled, Cross-Over Trial. *Clin. Gastroenterol. Hepatol. Off. Clin. Pr. J. Am. Gastroenterol. Assoc.* **2015**, *13*, 1604–1612.e3. [CrossRef]
51. Rosinach, M.; Fernández-Bañares, F.; Carrasco, A.; Ibarra, M.; Temiño, R.; Salas, A.; Esteve, M. Double-Blind Randomized Clinical Trial: Gluten versus Placebo Rechallenge in Patients with Lymphocytic Enteritis and Suspected Celiac Disease. *PLoS ONE* **2016**, *11*, e0157879. [CrossRef] [PubMed]
52. Carroccio, A.; D'Alcamo, A.; Iacono, G.; Soresi, M.; Iacobucci, R.; Arini, A.; Geraci, G.; Fayer, F.; Cavataio, F.; La Blasca, F.; et al. Persistence of Nonceliac Wheat Sensitivity, Based on Long-term Follow-up. *Gastroenterology* **2017**, *153*, 56–58.e3. [CrossRef] [PubMed]
53. Roncoroni, L.; Bascuñán, K.A.; Vecchi, M.; Doneda, L.; Bardella, M.T.; Lombardo, V.; Scricciolo, A.; Branchi, F.; Elli, L. Exposure to Different Amounts of Dietary Gluten in Patients with Non-Celiac Gluten Sensitivity (NCGS): An Exploratory Study. *Nutrients* **2019**, *11*, 136. [CrossRef] [PubMed]
54. Carroccio, A.; Brusca, I.; Mansueto, P.; Soresi, M.; D'Alcamo, A.; Ambrosiano, G.; Pepe, I.; Iacono, G.; Lospalluti, M.L.; La Chiusa, S.M.; et al. Fecal assays detect hypersensitivity to cow's milk protein and gluten in adults with irritable bowel syndrome. *Clin. Gastroenterol. Hepatol. Off. Clin. Pr. J. Am. Gastroenterol. Assoc.* **2011**, *9*, 956–971.e3. [CrossRef] [PubMed]

55. Carroccio, A.; Mansueto, P.; Iacono, G.; Soresi, M.; D'Alcamo, A.; Cavataio, F.; Brusca, I.; Florena, A.M.; Ambrosiano, G.; Seidita, A.; et al. Non-celiac wheat sensitivity diagnosed by double-blind placebo-controlled challenge: Exploring a new clinical entity. *Am. J. Gastroenterol.* **2012**, *107*, 1898–1907. [CrossRef]
56. Volta, U.; Tovoli, F.; Cicola, R.; Parisi, C.; Fabbri, A.; Piscaglia, M.; Fiorini, E.; Caio, G. Serological Tests in Gluten Sensitivity (Nonceliac Gluten Intolerance). *J. Clin. Gastroenterol.* **2012**, *46*, 680–685. [CrossRef]
57. Carroccio, A.; D'Alcamo, A.; Cavataio, F.; Soresi, M.; Seidita, A.; Sciumè, C.; Geraci, G.; Iacono, G.; Mansueto, P. High Proportions of People with Nonceliac Wheat Sensitivity Have Autoimmune Disease or Antinuclear Antibodies. *Gastroenterology* **2015**, *149*, 596–603.e1. [CrossRef]
58. Infantino, M.; Manfredi, M.; Meacci, F.; Grossi, V.; Severino, M.; Benucci, M.; Bellio, E.; Bellio, V.; Nucci, A.; Zolfanelli, F.; et al. Diagnostic accuracy of anti-gliadin antibodies in Non-Celiac Gluten Sensitivity (NCGS) patients. *Clin. Chim. Acta* **2015**, *451*, 135–141. [CrossRef]
59. Norsa, L.; Shamir, R.; Zevit, N.; Verduci, E.; Hartman, C.; Ghisleni, D.; Riva, E.; Giovannini, M. Cardiovascular disease risk factor profiles in children with celiac disease on gluten-free diets. *World J. Gastroenterol.* **2013**, *19*, 5658–5664. [CrossRef]
60. Jenkins, D.J.; Kendall, C.W.; Vidgen, E.; Augustin, L.S.; van Erk, M.; Geelen, A.; Parker, T.; Faulkner, D.; Vuksan, V.; Josse, R.G.; et al. High-protein diets in hyperlipidemia: Effect of wheat gluten on serum lipids, uric acid, and renal function. *Am. J. Clin. Nutr.* **2001**, *74*, 57–63. [CrossRef]
61. Jenkins, D.J.; Kendall, C.W.; Vuksan, V.; Augustin, L.S.; Mehling, C.; Parker, T.; Vidgen, E.; Lee, B.; Faulkner, D.; Seyler, H.; et al. Effect of wheat bran on serum lipids: Influence of particle size and wheat protein. *J. Am. Coll Nutr.* **1999**, *18*, 159–165. [CrossRef] [PubMed]
62. Lebwohl, B.; Cao, Y.; Zong, G.; Hu, F.B.; Green, P.H.R.; Neugut, A.I.; Rimm, E.B.; Sampson, L.; Dougherty, L.W.; Giovannucci, E.; et al. Long term gluten consumption in adults without celiac disease and risk of coronary heart disease: Prospective cohort study. *BMJ* **2017**, *357*, j1892. [CrossRef] [PubMed]
63. Niland, B.; Cash, B.D. Health Benefits and Adverse Effects of a Gluten-Free Diet in Non–Celiac Disease Patients. *Gastroenterol Hepatol.* **2018**, *14*, 82–91.
64. Vici, G.; Belli, L.; Biondi, M.; Polzonetti, V. Gluten free diet and nutrient deficiencies: A review. *Clin. Nutr. Edinb. Scotl.* **2016**, *35*, 1236–1241. [CrossRef] [PubMed]
65. Hallert, C.; Grant, C.; Grehn, S.; Grännö, C.; Hultén, S.; Midhagen, G.; Ström, M.; Svensson, H.; Valdimarsson, T. Evidence of poor vitamin status in coeliac patients on a gluten-free diet for 10 years. *Aliment. Pharm. Ther.* **2002**, *16*, 1333–1339. [CrossRef]
66. Tovoli, F.; Granito, A.; Negrini, G.; Guidetti, E.; Faggiano, C.; Bolondi, L. Long term effects of gluten-free diet in non-celiac wheat sensitivity. *Clin. Nutr. Edinb. Scotl.* **2019**, *38*, 357–363. [CrossRef] [PubMed]

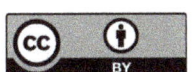

© 2019 by the authors. Licensee MDPI, Basel, Switzerland. This article is an open access article distributed under the terms and conditions of the Creative Commons Attribution (CC BY) license (http://creativecommons.org/licenses/by/4.0/).

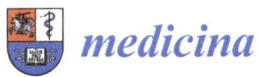

Review

Relevance of HLA-DQB1*02 Allele in the Genetic Predisposition of Children with Celiac Disease: Additional Cues from a Meta-Analysis

Cristina Capittini [1], Annalisa De Silvestri [1], Chiara Rebuffi [2], Carmine Tinelli [1] and Dimitri Poddighe [3,*]

- [1] Scientific Direction, Clinical Epidemiology and Biometric Unit, Fondazione IRCCS Policlinico San Matteo, 27100 Pavia, Italy; C.Capittini@smatteo.pv.it (C.C.); a.desilvestri@smatteo.pv.it (A.D.S.); ctinelli@smatteo.pv.it (C.T.)
- [2] Grant Office and Scientific Documentation Center, Fondazione IRCCS Policlinico San Matteo, 27100 Pavia, Italy; C.Rebuffi@smatteo.pv.it
- [3] Department of Medicine, Nazarbayev University School of Medicine, Nur-Sultan City 010000, Kazakhstan
- * Correspondence: dimitri.poddighe@nu.edu.kz; Tel.: +7-7172-694637

Received: 20 March 2019; Accepted: 14 May 2019; Published: 22 May 2019

Abstract: *Background and Objectives:* Celiac disease (CD) is a multifactorial immune-mediated disorder, triggered by the ingestion of gluten in genetically-predisposed subjects carrying MHC-DQ2 and -DQ8 heterodimers, which are encoded by four HLA-DQ allelic variants, overall. This meta-analysis aims at providing further epidemiological support to the predominant relevance of one specific allele, namely HLA-DQB1*02, in the predisposition and genetic risk of CD. *Materials and Methods:* We performed a search of MEDLINE/PubMed, Embase, Web of Science, and Scopus, retrieving all publications (case–control study, cross-sectional, and retrospective cohort study) on the association between HLA class II polymorphisms and first-degree relatives (FDRs) of children with CD. After a critical reading of the articles, two investigators independently performed data extraction according to the following inclusion criteria: HLA class II genes, any DQ and DR molecules, and CD diagnosed following the current clinical guidelines. A third participant was consulted for discussion to reach an agreement concerning discrepancies. *Results:* Our search strategy selected 14 studies as being eligible for inclusion, and those were submitted for data extraction and analysis. These studies were published between 1999 and 2016 and, collectively, enrolled 3063 FDRs. Positive and negative likelihood ratios (LR+ and LR−, respectively) for CD diagnosis, according to the presence of the HLA-DQ genotype coding a complete MHC-DQ2 and/or MHC-DQ8 molecules, were 1.449 (CI 1.279–1.642) and 0.187 (CI 0.096–0.362), respectively. If only the isolated presence of HLA-DQB1*02 allele is considered, the pooled estimation of LR+ was 1.659 (CI 1.302–2.155) and, importantly, the LR− still showed a very good discriminatory power of 0.195 (CI 0.068–0.558). *Conclusions:* Through our differential meta-analysis, comparing the presence of the genotype coding the full MHC-DQ2 and/or DQ8 molecules with the isolated presence of HLA-DQB1*02 allelic variant, we found that the LR− of the latter analysis maintained the same value. This observation, along with previous evidences, might be useful to consider potential cost-effective widened screening strategies for CD in children.

Keywords: celiac disease; children; HLA-DQB1*02; screening; first-degree relatives

1. Introduction

Celiac disease (CD) is a multifactorial immune-mediated disorder, triggered by the ingestion of gluten and other gluten-related proteins in genetically predisposed subjects. Importantly, the HLA-DQ alleles, coding α and β chains of the MHC-DQ2 and -DQ8 heterodimers, have been shown to be a necessary, but not sufficient, immunogenetic background for the development of CD. These HLA-DQ haplotypes have been estimated to contribute up to 25%–40% of the genetic risk for CD and have been reported to be present in around 35–40% of the general population in North America and Europe, where the prevalence of CD is close to 1% and, probably, even more if only the pediatric population is considered [1,2].

In particular, children are a vulnerable population with respect to the complications and long-term consequences of untreated CD, taking into account also their longer life-expectancy. Moreover, in addition to gastrointestinal symptoms, a considerable number of patients with CD present extra-gastrointestinal manifestations only (leading to under-diagnosis and/or significant diagnostic delays), and some patients may be completely asymptomatic, although they often report a subjective improvement after starting a gluten-free diet. Long-term complications of untreated CD are plausible, but there are still few studies addressing this specific issue [2–6].

All these epidemiological and clinical aspects have stimulated the scientific debate about the possibility to implement a wider screening strategy to identify CD patients, especially in children. Indeed, the screening approach by active case-finding, limited to the first-degree relatives (FDRs) of CD patients and children affected with other autoimmune diseases or chromosomal aberrations (known to be statistically associated with CD), was only partially effective as most asymptomatic or mildly symptomatic patients have no clear risk factors and, thus, cannot be detected [7,8]. However, extending the serological screening to all children and repeating it at several ages in childhood, is not a sustainable approach and, therefore, alternative strategies must be sought.

It is well known that HLA-DQ genotyping is useful to ascertain the susceptibility to CD with very high—if not absolute—discriminatory power. Indeed, it is very unlikely that individuals who do not carry any specific HLA-DQ alleles, coding MHC-DQ2 (HLA-DQA1*05 + HLA-DQB1*02) and MHC-DQ8 (HLA-DQA1*03 + HLA-DQB1*03:02) heterodimers, can develop CD [1,8]. Such a knowledge resulted to be very useful in the diagnostic approach to some complex cases (e.g. patients with antibody deficiencies) and, importantly, was able to avoid the duodenal biopsies in those children fulfilling some specific clinical and serological criteria, according to the ESPGHAN (European Society for Pediatric Gastroenterology, Hepatology and Nutrition) guidelines, published in 2012 [9]. Recently, several groups started to investigate the possibility to take advantage of specific HLA-DQ genetic analyses for a potential multi-step approach to extend the screening for CD to children who are not considered to be at higher risk, as defined above. That may be feasible through a reduction of the costs for the genetic analysis, compared to the high-resolution HLA genotyping. For this purpose, one contributing factor may be limiting the genetic analysis to specific CD-predisposed HLA-DQ alleles and, in particular, to the HLA-DQB1*02 allele, which plays a relevant role in CD genetic predisposition, according to the risk gradient showed in Figure 1 [8,10–12]. Through this meta-analysis, we aim at providing further epidemiological support to this potential approach.

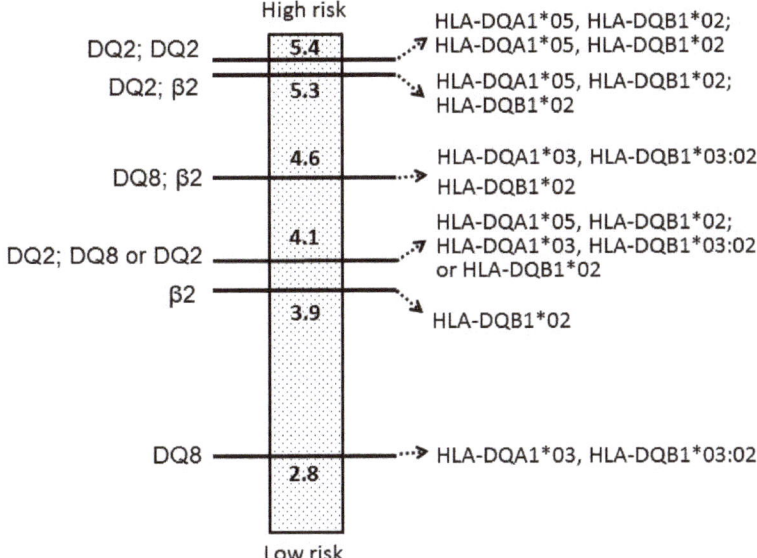

Figure 1. HLA-DQ risk gradient for Celiac Disease according to the odds-ratio (OR) values from our previous meta-analysis (modified from De Silvestri et al.).

2. Materials and Methods

2.1. Protocol

This work was written according to PRISMA guidelines [13], as described in Figure 2. Through this meta-analysis, we aimed at quantitatively evaluating the association between HLA-DQ polymorphisms and the susceptibility to CD in FDRs of pediatric CD patients.

2.2. Search Strategy

We performed a search of PubMed, EMBASE, Web of Science, and Scopus, retrieving all publications (case-control study, cross-sectional, and retrospective cohort study) on the association between HLA class II polymorphisms and first-degree relatives (FDRs) of CD children. We searched all articles published up to September 2018 in several languages (English, French, German, Italian, Portuguese, and Spanish).

We performed the search strategy using a free-text search (keywords) and thesaurus descriptors search (MeSH and Emtree) for each concept, adapted by a trained librarian for all the selected databases. In detail, an expert librarian performed the search by using the following terms: ("celiac disease" [MeSH] OR "celiac disease" [tiab] OR "coeliac disease" [tiab]) AND ("Histocompatibility Antigens Class II" [Mesh] OR "Histocompatibility Antigens Class II" [tiab]) AND ("nuclear family" [mesh] OR relative* [tiab] OR sibling* [tiab] OR parent* [tiab]) AND ("mass screening" [mesh] OR screening [tiab] OR prevalence[tiab] OR "Prevalence" [Mesh] OR "Predictive Value of Tests" [Mesh] OR "predictive value" [tiab]). In Embase, the search used the following terms: ('celiac disease'/exp OR 'celiac disease':ti,ab OR 'coeliac disease':ti,ab) AND ('HLA antigen class 2'/exp OR "Histocompatibility Antigens Class II":ti,ab) AND ('nuclear family'/exp OR relative*:ti,ab OR sibling*:ti,ab OR parent*:ti,ab) AND ('screening'/exp OR screening:ti,ab OR 'Prevalence'/exp OR prevalence:ti,ab OR 'predictive value'/exp OR 'predictive value':ti,ab). In Web of Science, the search used the following terms: ("celiac disease" OR "coeliac disease") AND HLA AND (relative* OR sibling* OR parent*) AND (screening OR prevalence OR "predictive value"). In Scopus, the search used the following terms: "celiac disease" OR "coeliac disease" AND HLA AND (relative* OR sibling* OR parent*) AND (screening OR prevalence OR "predictive value").

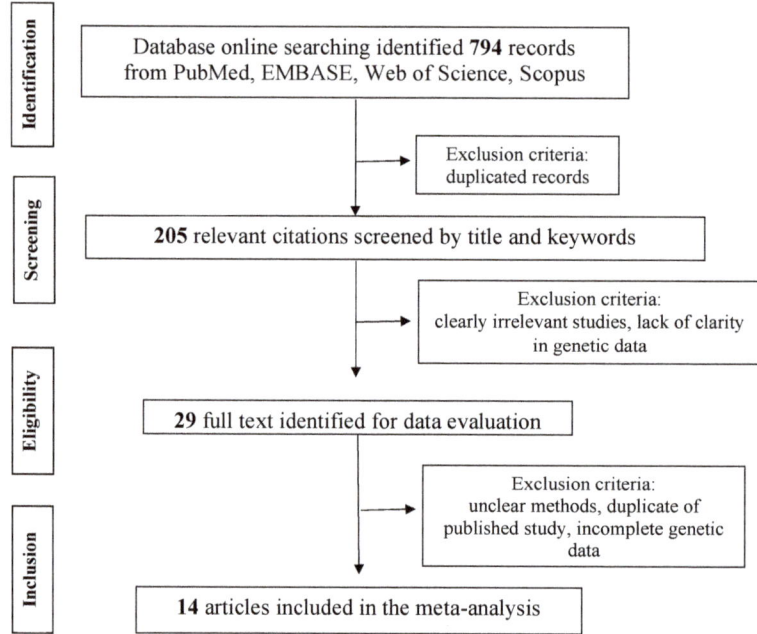

Figure 2. Flow diagram of the study following the PRISMA guidelines.

2.3. Data Extraction

After a critical reading of the articles, two investigators independently performed data extraction according to the following inclusion criteria: HLA class II genes, any DQ and DR molecules, and celiac disease diagnosed following the clinical criteria set by Meeuwisse (1969–1970), Walker-Smith et al. (1990–2012), and Husby et al. (2012 ESPGHAN guidelines) [9,14,15]. The third participant was consulted for discussion to reach an agreement concerning discrepancies.

2.4. Data Synthesis and Meta-Analysis

STATA 14.2 (StataCorp., College Station, TX, USA) and METADISC 1.4 were used for statistical analysis to perform meta-analysis the [16]. Heterogeneity was checked through the χ^2-test and the I-squared statistics [17]. The criteria for identification of heterogeneity were p values less than 0.10 for the χ^2-test and an I-squared value greater than 50%. When there was no statistical evidence for heterogeneity in effect sizes, we used the fixed-effect model to analyze odds ratios (ORs) or relative risks in FDRs. When significant heterogeneity was identified, we used the random-effects model (REM) and explored sources of significant heterogeneity [18,19].

We considered all studies including subjects analyzed for both the HLA-DQA1*05 and HLA-DQB1*02 alleles (coding the DQ2 molecule) and/or for the HLA-DQA1*03 and HLA-DQB1*03:02 alleles (coding the DQ8 molecule). For each selected study, we calculated sensitivity, specificity, positive likelihood ratio (LR+), and negative likelihood ratio (LR−) to develop CD. In order to produce clinically useful statistics, we calculated the pooled LR+ and LR− values. For all estimated values, we provided the 95% confidence interval (CI).

3. Results

3.1. Study Selection

Our search strategy yielded 794 papers for consideration. Following elimination of duplicates, 205 titles and/or abstracts were reviewed. Of these, 176 were excluded and, among the remaining 29 full-text manuscripts, 14 studies were deemed eligible for inclusion and were submitted to data extraction and analysis (refer to Figure 2). These studies were published between 1999 and 2016 and, collectively, enrolled 3063 FDRs. In detail, our analysis included three studies from India, two studies each from Chile, Italy, and Spain, and 1 study each from Brazil, Cuba, Jordan, Finland, and the USA [20–33].

Among the 3063 FDRs, 1720 patients were MHC-DQ2 or -DQ8 carriers, but only 352 were diagnosed with CD; among these, 337 patients were MHC-DQ2 or -DQ8 carriers. Thus, the prevalence of CD among FDRs was around 11.5% (CI 10–12).

3.2. Study Quality

The quality of selected studies, in terms of laboratory methods, methods description, statistical methodology and clinical features, was assessed according to PRISMA standards and resulted to be appropriate.

3.3. Meta-Analysis According to the Complete MHC-DQ2 and/or DQ8 Genotype

In our meta-analysis, we expressed these parameters as positive and negative likelihood ratios (LR+ and LR−, respectively) for CD, according to the presence of the HLA-DQ genotype coding complete MHC-DQ2 and/or MHC-DQ8 molecules. The pooled estimation of LR+ was 1.449 (CI 1.279–1.642), whereas LR− was 0.187 (0.096–0.362). While this HLA-DQ background is known to provide a low specificity (Table 1), its presence is actually characterized with very high sensitivity for CD, showing a good discriminatory power between genetically predisposed CD (not necessarily affected) patients and those who will not develop CD, as shown in Table 2.

Table 1. Positive likelihood ratio (LR+) of MHC-DQ2 and/or -DQ8 genotype in first-degree relatives (FDRs) of pediatric celiac disease (CD) patients (Heterogeneity $\chi^2 = 132.54$ (d.f. = 13), $p < 0.001$; Inconsistency (I-squared) = 90.2%; and estimate of between-study variance (Tau-squared) = 0.0455).

Summary—Positive Likelihood Ratio (Random Effects Model)				
Study (Year)	Country	LR+	95% Conf. Interval	% Weight
Araya et al. (2015)	Chile	1.008	0.749–1.357	5.92
Araya et al. (2000)	Chile	7.557	4.475–12.762	3.47
Bonamico et al. (2006)	Italy	1.779	1.572–2.014	8.20
Cintado et al. (2006)	Cuba	1.054	0.809–1.372	6.38
Elakawi et al. (2010)	Jordan	1.487	1.061–2.084	5.40
Farre et al. (1999)	Spain	1.563	1.317–1.854	7.64
Karinen et al. (2006)	Finland		1.008–1.255	8.35
Martins et al. (2010)	Brazil	1.691	1.393–2.052	7.35
Megiorni et al. (2009)	Italy	1.707	1.590–1.832	8.67
Mishra et al. (2016)	India	1.304	1.126–1.511	7.94
Rubio-Tapia et al. (2010)	USA	1.413	1.302–1.533	8.59
Singla et al. (2016)	India	1.148	1.040–1.268	8.45
Srivastava et al. (2010)	India	1.063	0.783–1.443	5.82
Vaquero et al. (2014)	Spain	1.530	1.309–1.789	7.83
(REM) pooled LR+		1.449	1.279–1.642	

Table 2. Negative likelihood ratio (LR−) of MHC-DQ2 and/or -DQ8 genotype in FDRs of pediatric CD patients (Heterogeneity χ^2 = 20.34 (d.f. = 13), p = 0.087; inconsistency (I-squared) = 36.1%; and estimate of between-study variance (Tau-squared) = 0.4949).

Summary—Negative Likelihood Ratio (Random Effects Model)				
Study (Year)	Country	LR−	95% Conf. Interval	% Weight
Araya et al. (2015)	Chile	0.933	0.065–13.461	4.86
Araya et al. (2000)	Chile	0.081	0.006–1.178	4.86
Bonamico et al. (2006)	Italy	0.107	0.028–0.416	11.74
Cintado et al. (2006)	Cuba	0.641	0.041–10.017	4.64
Elakawi et al. (2010)	Jordan	0.217	0.015–3.170	4.83
Farre et al. (1999)	Spain	0.108	0.007–1.636	4.72
Karinen et al. (2006)	Finland	0.526	0.265–1.044	18.52
Martins et al. (2010)	Brazil	0.158	0.024–1.054	7.99
Megiorni et al. (2009)	Italy	0.044	0.006–0.310	7.73
Mishra et al. (2016)	India	0.188	0.047–0.757	11.43
Rubio-Tapia et al. (2010)	USA	0.042	0.003–0.656	4.61
Singla et al. (2016)	India	0.173	0.011–2.730	4.61
Srivastava et al. (2010)	India	0.652	0.045–9.460	4.85
Vaquero et al. (2014)	Spain	0.043	0.003–0.674	4.60
(REM) pooled LR−		0.187	0.096–0.362	

3.4. Meta-Analysis According to the Isolated Presence of HLA-DQB1*02 Allele

DQB1*02 sensitivity was 0.938 (CI 0.891–0.968) and specificity was 0.425 (CI 0.400–0.451). We meta-analyzed the LR+ and LR− of FDRs according to the presence of the DQB1*02 allele. The pooled estimate of LR+ was 1.659 (CI 1.302–2.155) (Table 3), whereas LR− showed a good discriminatory power of 0.195 (CI 0.068–0.558) (Table 4).

Table 3. Positive likelihood ratio (LR+) related to the DQB1*02 allele in FDRs of pediatric CD patients (Heterogeneity χ^2 = 89.02 (d.f. = 6), p < 0.001; inconsistency (I-squared) = 93.3%; and estimate of between-study variance (Tau-squared) = 0.0906).

Summary—Positive Likelihood Ratio (Random Effects Model)			
Study (Year)	LR+	95% Conf. Interval	% Weight
Araya et al. (2015)	7.557	4.475–12.762	9.44
Cintado et al. (2006)	1.054	0.809–1.372	14.07
Elakawi et al. (2010)	1.487	1.061–2.084	12.72
Farre et al. (1999)	1.563	1.317–1.854	15.58
Karinen et al. (2006)	1.125	1.008–1.255	16.32
Martins et al. (2010)	1.691	1.393–2.052	15.24
Megiorni et al. (2009)	1.707	1.590–1.832	16.64
(REM) pooled LR+	1.659	1.302–2.115	

Table 4. Negative likelihood ratio (LR−) related to the DQB1*02 allele in FDRs of pediatric CD patients (Heterogeneity χ^2 = 12.06 (d.f. = 6), p = 0.061; inconsistency (I-squared) = 50.2%; and estimate of between-study variance (Tau-squared) = 0.9053).

Summary—Negative Likelihood Ratio (Random Effects Model)			
Study (year)	LR−	95% Conf. Interval	% Weight
Araya et al. (2015)	0.081	0.006–1.178	10.43
Cintado et al. (2006)	0.641	0.041–10.017	10.03
Elakawi et al. (2010)	0.217	0.015–3.170	10.38
Farre et al. (1999)	0.108	0.007–1.636	10.18
Karinen et al. (2006)	0.526	0.265–1.044	28.05
Martins et al. (2010)	0.158	0.024–1.054	15.66
Megiorni et al. (2009)	0.044	0.006–0.310	15.26
(REM) pooled LR−	0.195	0.068–0.558	

4. Discussion

This meta-analysis confirmed the very high negative predictive value associated with the absence of the HLA-DQ genotype, coding MHC-DQ2 and/or -DQ8, as regards the risk to developing CD. This long-established knowledge has been exploited to complete and/or refine the diagnostic work-up of patients suspected to be affected with CD, but having doubtful histopathological findings or concomitant diseases that can impair the reliability of the serological screening (e.g., IgA deficiency, common variable immunodeficiency) [22,34]. More recently, this genetic analysis has been included in the ESPGHAN guidelines to diagnose CD without performing any duodenal biopsy in children with consistent symptoms, high-titer of anti-tTG IgA, and EMA positivity [9]. However, beyond these practical conditions, the poor positive predictive value of being carrier of MHC-DQ2 and/or -DQ8 heterodimers, cannot provide any additional usefulness to the diagnosis of CD, in addition to confirming the necessary genetic predisposition.

Additionally, in this meta-analysis we separately analyzed the positive and negative predictive values (expressed as positive and negative LRs, respectively) related to the presence and absence of the HLA-DQB1*02 allele. Recently, Megiorni et al. reviewed the role of HLA-DQA1 and HLA-DQB1 in the predisposition to CD. They described a risk gradient whereby patients who are DQ2/DQ8 heterozygous and DQ2 homozygous showed a very high risk and, to follow, there were patients who were DQ8 homozygous, DQ8 heterozygous, along with DQ2 heterozygous, and, then, people carrying a double dose of DQB1*02 only [35]. Importantly, these latter patients showed a similar risk of CD as the previous categories, although they did not carry the complete MHC-DQ2 or MHC-DQ8 heterodimer.

Recently, a previous meta-analysis by our group supported this observation: we showed that a double dose of HLA-DQB1*02 was associated with the highest risk to develop pediatric CD (OR > 5), regardless of other HLA-DQ alleles. Moreover, even a single "dose" of HLA-DQB1*02 was associated with a relatively high risk (OR around 4) for pediatric CD. Basically, our statistical analysis suggested that children carrying only one HLA-DQB1*02 copy (without any other allele related to MHC-DQ2 or MHC-DQ8 molecules) have a similar predisposition/risk to become celiac as children expressing the full MHC-DQ2 and/or MHC-DQ8 molecules [8]. Accordingly, the original research by Megiorni et al., including 437 Italian children with CD and 551 controls, described a disease risk of 1:26 for children being homozygous for HLA-DQB1*02 (despite the absence of the other genes coding for DQ2 or DQ8); children being double heterozygous DQ2/DQ8, heterozygous DQ2 with double dose HLA-DQB1*02, and DQ8 heterozygous along with one HLA-DQB1*02 allele, showed a disease risk of 1:7, 1:10, and 1:24, respectively [28]. Therefore, all these studies suggested a major relevance of HLA-DQB1*02 allele in conferring the risk to develop pediatric CD, rather than the expression of the full MHC-DQ2 and/or -DQ8 heterodimers. Moreover, a risk gradient according to the dose ("single" or "double" copy of HLA-DQB1*02) has been evidenced.

Through our differential meta-analysis, comparing the presence of the full MHC-DQ2 and/or DQ8 genotypes and the isolated presence of HLA-DQB1*02 allelic variant, we found that the negative LR (namely the negative predictive value) was basically the same (0.187 vs. 0.195). Unfortunately, we could not obtain enough data to perform the same statistical analysis considering the HLA-DQB1*03:02 solely, as its frequency in the general population and CD patients is much lower compared to the HLA-DQB1*02 allele.

However, some molecular studies supported this concept that HLA-DQB1*02 may play a major role in the interaction between class II MHC molecule and the gliadin-derived peptide to be presented to T-lymphocytes, in order to trigger all immunological events involved in the pathogenesis of CD [36]. Indeed, the high content of proline and glutamine residues of MHC-DQ2-restricted gliadin epitopes resulted to be fundamental for the interaction and binding to the class II MHC molecules. One research showed that some specific DQ2 β chain residues, participating in the formation of the peptide-binding cleft (particularly Arg-β70 and Lys-β71 of β chain encoded by HLA-DQB1*02), are mainly responsible for the interaction with several residues of the gliadin epitope and, thus, may be critical to the CD predisposition [37].

Previously, we showed that 90–95% of CD children seem to carry at least a single copy of HLA-DQB1*02, regardless of the remaining HLA-DQ genotype [8]. Moreover, we supported this finding in our monocentric case series, including 269 children with CD, where >97% of all these CD children possessed at least one copy of HLA-DQB1*02 allele in their individual genotype [38]. Here, we looked at the HLA-DQ asset in the FDRs of pediatric CD patients and we found that the almost absolute negative LR was maintained, even when we considered only HLA-DQB1*02 in our analysis. This comparison suggests that the absence of this allele from the individual HLA-DQ genotype might rule out any individual predisposition to develop CD, as well as the analysis of the full genotype coding complete MHC-DQ2/DQ8 heterodimer(s) can do, without any significant decrease in the negative predictive value for CD.

These observations may contribute to the debate about the potential and cost-effective implementation of wider or mass-screening strategies for CD in children. Indeed, a low-cost HLA-DQ analysis, specific for CD predisposition, may allow to select those 30–40% of children who really deserve the serological screening [39–41].

The qualitative analysis to screen the presence of HLA-DQB1*02 in order to establish the genetic predisposition in the general population, may be one potential approach, and the complete HLA-DQ genotyping might be reserved to children with clinical suspicion, if needed [8,10,12]. Of course, further epidemiological, clinical and genetic researches are required in order to establish if this approach may be appropriate, feasible and cost-effective. However, other researchers considered a potential multi-step approach to screen CD, starting from the analysis of the specific genetic predisposition to CD through low-cost molecular methods. Recently, Verma et al. proposed a rapid HLA-DQ typing method to identify subjects genetically susceptible to CD. Basically, they performed a PCR through a kit containing the primers for the HLA-DQ target alleles only, on blood samples from CD patients, FDRs and controls. They could show an excellent concordance with the results obtained through conventional high-resolution HLA-DQ typing, in terms of presence or absence of HLA-DQ2 and HLA-DQ8 alleles [11]. The implementation of cost-effective screening strategies may be very helpful, not only in Western countries (where CD has been widely studied and described), but also in developing countries, where a number of health system-related barriers have not permitted an evidence-based approach to the diagnosis of CD, yet [42–44].

Therefore, if our observations will be supported by further and independent studies, those may represent an additional contribution to reduce the cost of a targeted genetic analysis for CD.

5. Conclusions

Through a differential meta-analysis, comparing the presence of the genotype coding the full MHC-DQ2 and/or DQ8 molecules and the isolated presence of HLA-DQB1*02 allelic variant, we found that the LR− of the latter analysis maintained the same value. This observation, along with the previous evidences, might be useful to consider potential cost-effective widened screening strategies for CD in children.

Author Contributions: D.P. and C.C. conceived and wrote this manuscript; A.D.S. and C.T. analyzed data; C.R. made the systematic search; A.D.S. collected data and made the tables; C.C. made the figures; D.P. and C.T. provided substantial intellectual contribution; C.C., A.D.S., C.R., C.T., D.P. approved the manuscript.

Funding: This work was supported by research project number 870-rcr2016-50 from IRCCS Foundation Policlinico San Matteo (Pavia, Italy).

Conflicts of Interest: The authors declare no conflict of interest.

References

1. Lindfors, K.; Ciacci, C.; Kurppa, K.; Lundin, K.E.A.; Makharia, G.K.; Mearin, M.L.; Murray, J.A.; Verdu, E.F.; Kaukinen, K. Coeliac disease. *Nat. Rev. Dis. Primers* **2019**, *5*, 3. [CrossRef] [PubMed]
2. Lebwohl, B.; Sanders, D.S.; Green, P.H.R. Coeliac disease. *Lancet* **2018**, *391*, 70–81. [CrossRef]
3. Ludvigsson, J.F. Mortality and malignancy in celiac disease. *Gastrointest. Endosc. Clin. N. Am.* **2012**, *22*, 705–722. [CrossRef]
4. Abdul Sultan, A.; Crooks, C.J.; Card, T.; Tata, L.J.; Fleming, K.M.; West, J. Causes of death in people with coeliac disease in England compared with the general population: A competing risk analysis. *Gut* **2015**, *64*, 1220–1226. [CrossRef] [PubMed]
5. Paarlahti, P.; Kurppa, K.; Ukkola, A.; Collin, P.; Huhtala, H.; Mäki, M.; Kaukinen, K. Predictors of persistent symptoms and reduced quality of life in treated coeliac disease patients: A large cross-sectional study. *BMC Gastroenterol.* **2013**, *13*, 75. [CrossRef]
6. Stordal, K.; Bakken, I.J.; Suren, P. Epidemiology of coeliac disease and comorbidity in Norwegian children. *J. Pediatr. Gastroenterol. Nutr.* **2013**, *57*, 467–471. [CrossRef] [PubMed]
7. Bjorck, S.; Brundin, C.; Lorinc, E.; Lynch, K.F.; Agardh, D. Screening detects a high proportion of celiac disease in young HLA-genotyped children. *J. Pediatr. Gastroenterol. Nutr.* **2010**, *50*, 49–53. [CrossRef]
8. De Silvestri, A.; Capittini, C.; Poddighe, D.; Valsecchi, C.; Marseglia, G.; Tagliacarne, S.C.; Scotti, V.; Rebuffi, C.; Pasi, A.; Martinetti, M.; Tinelli, C. HLA-DQ genetics in children with celiac disease: A meta-analysis suggesting a two-step genetic screening procedure starting with HLA-DQ β chains. *Pediatr. Res.* **2018**, *83*, 564–572. [CrossRef]
9. Husby, S.; Koletzko, S.; Korponay-Szabó, I.R.; Mearin, M.L.; Phillips, A.; Shamir, R.; Troncone, R.; Giersiepen, K.; Branski, D.; Catassi, C.; et al. ESPGHAN Working Group on Coeliac Disease Diagnosis; ESPGHAN Gastroenterology Committee; European Society for Pediatric Gastroenterology, Hepatology, and Nutrition. European Society for Pediatric Gastroenterology, Hepatology, and Nutrition guidelines for the diagnosis of coeliac disease. *J. Pediatr. Gastroenterol. Nutr.* **2012**, *54*, 136–160. [PubMed]
10. Poddighe, D. Individual screening strategy for pediatric celiac disease. *Eur. J. Pediatr.* **2018**, *177*, 1871. [CrossRef] [PubMed]
11. Verma, A.K.; Singh, A.; Gatti, S.; Lionetti, E.; Galeazzi, T.; Monachesi, C.; Franceschini, E.; Ahuja, V.; Catassi, C.; Makharia, G.K. Validation of a novel single-drop rapid human leukocyte antigen-DQ2/-DQ8 typing method to identify subjects susceptible to celiac disease. *JGH Open* **2018**, *2*, 311–316. [CrossRef]
12. Poddighe, D. Relevance of HLA-DQB1*02 allele in predisposing to Coeliac Disease. *Int. J. Immunogenet.* **2019**, in press. [CrossRef]
13. Moher, D.; Liberati, A.; Tetzlaff, J.; Altman, D.G.; PRISMA Group. Preferred reporting items for systematic reviews and meta-analyses: The PRISMA statement. *J. Clin. Epidemiol.* **2009**, *62*, 1006–1012. [CrossRef]
14. Meeuwisse, G.W. Round table discussion. Diagnostic criteria in coeliac disease. *Acta Paediatr. Scand.* **1970**, *59*, 461–463.
15. Walker-Smith, J.A.; Guandalini, S.; Schmitz, J. Revised criteria for diagnosis of coeliac disease. *Arch. Dis. Child.* **1990**, *65*, 909–911.

16. Zamora, J.; Abraira, V.; Muriel, A.; Khan, K.; Coomarasamy, A. Meta-DiSc: A software for metaanalysis of test accuracy data. *BMC Med. Res. Methodol.* **2006**, *6*, 31. [CrossRef] [PubMed]
17. Higgins, J.P.; Thompson, S.G. Quantifying heterogeneity in a meta-analysis. *Stat. Med.* **2002**, *21*, 1539–1558. [CrossRef] [PubMed]
18. Der Simonian, R.; Laird, N. Meta-analysis in clinical trials. *Control. Clin. Trials* **1986**, *7*, 177–188. [CrossRef]
19. Higgins, J.P.T.; Green, S. Cochrane Handbook for Systematic Reviews of Interventions, Version 5.1.0 (updated March 2011). The Cochrane Collaboration. Available online: http://www.cochrane-handbook.org (accessed on 1 March 2015).
20. Araya, M.; Oyarzun, A.; Lucero, Y.; Espinosa, N.; Pérez-Bravo, F. DQ2, DQ7 and DQ8 Distribution and Clinical Manifestations in Celiac Cases and Their First-Degree Relatives. *Nutrients* **2015**, *7*, 4955–4965. [CrossRef] [PubMed]
21. Araya, M.; Mondragón, A.; Pérez-Bravo, F.; Roessler, J.L.; Alarcón, T.; Rios, G.; Bergenfreid, C. Celiac disease in a Chilean population carrying Amerindian traits. *J. Pediatr. Gastroenterol. Nutr.* **2000**, *31*, 381–386. [CrossRef]
22. Bonamico, M.; Ferri, M.; Mariani, P.; Nenna, R.; Thanasi, E.; Luparia, R.P.; Picarelli, A.; Magliocca, F.M.; Mora, B.; Bardella, M.T.; Verrienti, A.; et al. Serologic and genetic markers of celiac disease: A sequential study in the screening of first degree relatives. *J. Pediatr. Gastroenterol. Nutr.* **2006**, *42*, 150–154. [CrossRef]
23. Cintado, A.; Sorell, L.; Galván, J.A.; Martínez, L.; Castañeda, C.; Fragoso, T.; Camacho, H.; Ferrer, A.; Companioni, O.; Benitez, J.; et al. HLA DQA1*0501 and DQB1*02 in Cuban celiac patients. *Hum. Immunol.* **2006**, *67*, 639–642. [CrossRef]
24. El-Akawi, Z.J.; Al-Hattab, D.M.; Migdady, M.A. Frequency of HLA-DQA1*0501 and DQB1*0201 alleles in patients with coeliac disease, their first-degree relatives and controls in Jordan. *Ann. Trop. Paediatr.* **2010**, *30*, 305–309. [CrossRef] [PubMed]
25. Farré, C.; Humbert, P.; Vilar, P.; Varea, V.; Aldeguer, X.; Carnicer, J.; Carballo, M.; Gassull, M.A. Serological markers and HLA-DQ2 haplotype among first-degree relatives of celiac patients. *Dig. Dis. Sci.* **1999**, *44*, 2344–2349. [CrossRef] [PubMed]
26. Karinen, H.; Kärkkäinen, P.; Pihlajamäki, J.; Janatuinen, E.; Heikkinen, M.; Julkunen, R.; Kosma, V.M.; Naukkarinen, A.; Laakso, M. HLA genotyping is useful in the evaluation of the risk for coeliac disease in the 1st-degree relatives of patients with coeliac disease. *Scand. J. Gastroenterol.* **2006**, *41*, 1299–1304. [CrossRef]
27. Martins, R.C.; Gandolfi, L.; Modelli, I.C.; Almeida, R.C.; Castro, L.C.; Pratesi, R. Serologic screening and genetic testing among brazilian patients with celiac disease and their first degree relatives. *Arq. Gastroenterol.* **2010**, *47*, 257–262. [CrossRef]
28. Megiorni, F.; Mora, B.; Bonamico, M.; Barbato, M.; Nenna, R.; Maiella, G.; Lulli, P.; Mazzilli, MC. HLA-DQ and risk gradient for celiac disease. *Hum. Immunol.* **2009**, *70*, 55–59. [CrossRef]
29. Mishra, A.; Prakash, S.; Kaur, G.; Sreenivas, V.; Ahuja, V.; Gupta, S.D.; Makharia, G.K. Prevalence of celiac disease among first-degree relatives of Indian celiac disease patients. *Dig. Liver Dis.* **2016**, *48*, 255–259. [CrossRef]
30. Rubio-Tapia, A.; Van Dyke, C.T.; Lahr, B.D.; Zinsmeister, A.R.; El-Youssef, M.; Moore, S.B.; Bowman, M.; Burgart, L.J.; Melton III, L.J.; Murray, J.A. Predictors of family risk for celiac disease: A population-based study. *Clin. Gastroenterol. Hepatol.* **2008**, *6*, 983–987. [CrossRef]
31. Singla, S.; Kumar, P.; Singh, P.; Kaur, G.; Rohtagi, A.; Choudhury, M. HLA Profile of Celiac Disease among First-Degree Relatives from a Tertiary Care Center in North India. *Ind. J. Pediatr.* **2016**, *83*, 1248–1252. [CrossRef]
32. Srivastava, A.; Yachha, S.K.; Mathias, A.; Parveen, F.; Poddar, U.; Agrawal, S. Prevalence, human leukocyte antigen typing and strategy for screening among Asian first-degree relatives of children with celiac disease. *J. Gastroenterol. Hepatol.* **2010**, *25*, 319–324. [CrossRef]
33. Vaquero, L.; Caminero, A.; Nuñez, A.; Hernando, M.; Iglesias, C.; Casqueiro, J.; Vivas, S. Coeliac disease screening in first-degree relatives on the basis of biopsy and genetic risk. *Eur. J. Gastroenterol. Hepatol.* **2014**, *26*, 263–267. [CrossRef]
34. Dorn, S.D.; Matchar, D.B. Cost-effectiveness analysis of strategies for diagnosing celiac disease. *Dig. Dis. Sci.* **2008**, *53*, 680–688. [CrossRef] [PubMed]
35. Megiorni, F.; Pizzuti, A. HLA-DQA1 and HLA-DQB1 in Celiac disease predisposition: Practical implications of the HLA molecular typing. *J. Biomed. Sci.* **2012**, *19*, 88. [CrossRef]

36. Vader, W.; Stepniak, D.; Kooy, Y.; Mearin, L.; Thompson, A.; van Rood, J.J.; Spaenij, L.; Koning, F. The HLA-DQ2 gene dose effect in celiac disease is directly related to the magnitude and breadth of gluten specific T cell responses. *Proc. Natl. Acad. Sci. USA* **2003**, *100*, 12390–12395. [CrossRef]
37. Sollid, L.M. Coeliac disease: Dissecting a complex inflammatory disorder. *Nat. Rev. Immunol.* **2002**, *2*, 647–655. [CrossRef]
38. Poddighe, D.; Capittini, C.; Gaviglio, I.; Brambilla, I.; Marseglia, G.L. HLA-DQB1*02 allele in children with Celiac Disease: Potential usefulness for screening strategies. *Int. J. Immunogenet.* **2019**, in press. [CrossRef]
39. Fernández-Fernández, S.; Borrell, B.; Cilleruelo, M.L.; Tabares, A.; Jiménez-Jiménez, J.; Rayo, A.I.; Perucho, T.; García-García, M.L. Prevalence of Celiac Disease in a Long-Term Study of a Spanish At-Genetic-Risk Cohort from the General Population. *J. Pediatr. Gastroenterol. Nutr.* **2019**, *68*, 364–370. [CrossRef]
40. Cilleruelo, M.L.; Fernández-Fernández, S.; Jiménez-Jiménez, J.; Rayo, A.I.; de Larramendi, C.H. Prevalence and Natural History of Celiac Disease in a Cohort of At-risk Children. *J. Pediatr. Gastroenterol. Nutr.* **2016**, *62*, 739–745. [CrossRef] [PubMed]
41. Wessels, M.M.S.; de Rooij, N.; Roovers, L.; Verhage, J.; de Vries, W.; Mearin, M.L. Towards an individual screening strategy for first-degree relatives of celiac patients. *Eur. J. Pediatr.* **2018**, *177*, 1585–1592. [CrossRef]
42. Makharia, G.K.; Catassi, C. Celiac Disease in Asia. *Gastroenterol. Clin. N. Am.* **2019**, *48*, 101–113.
43. Poddighe, D.; Rakhimzhanova, M.; Marchenko, Y.; Catassi, C. Pediatric Celiac Disease in Central and East Asia: Current Knowledge and Prevalence. *Medicina* **2019**, *55*, 11. [CrossRef]
44. Singh, P.; Arora, A.; Strand, T.A.; Leffler, DA.; Catassi, C.; Green, P.H.; Kelly, C.P.; Ahuja, V.; Makharia, G.K. Global Prevalence of Celiac Disease: Systematic Review and Meta-analysis. *Clin. Gastroenterol. Hepatol.* **2018**, *16*, 823–836. [CrossRef]

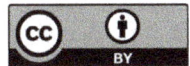

© 2019 by the authors. Licensee MDPI, Basel, Switzerland. This article is an open access article distributed under the terms and conditions of the Creative Commons Attribution (CC BY) license (http://creativecommons.org/licenses/by/4.0/).

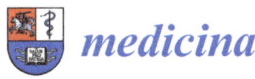

Review

Gluten Vehicle and Placebo for Non-Celiac Gluten Sensitivity Assessment

Oscar Gerardo Figueroa-Salcido [1], Noé Ontiveros [2,*] and Francisco Cabrera-Chavez [1,*]

1. Nutrition Sciences Academic Unit, Autonomous University of Sinaloa, Cedros y Calle Sauces S/N, Fraccionamiento Los Fresnos, Culiacán 80019, Sinaloa, Mexico; gerardofs95@hotmail.com
2. Division of Sciences and Engineering, Department of Chemical, Biological, and Agricultural Sciences (DC-QB), University of Sonora, Navojoa 85880, Sonora, Mexico
* Correspondence: noe.ontiveros@unison.mx (N.O.); fcabrera@uas.edu.mx (F.C.-C.)

Received: 5 April 2019; Accepted: 23 April 2019; Published: 26 April 2019

Abstract: Non-celiac gluten sensitivity (NCGS) is a syndrome characterized by gastrointestinal and extraintestinal manifestations triggered after gluten ingestion in the absence of celiac disease and wheat allergy. Because of the lack of biomarkers for NCGS diagnosis, the cornerstone for its assessment is a single- or double-blind placebo-controlled (DBPC) gluten challenge. However, there are some non-standardized points in the diagnostic approach proposed by the experts. This complicate comparisons among the results published by different research groups. The gluten vehicle and placebo must be indistinguishable from each other, which entails sensory and technological evaluations of the designed gluten vehicle and placebo products. At the moment, there is no standardized method for the preparation of the gluten vehicle and placebo for carrying out DBPC gluten challenges for NCGS assessment. This review focuses on the challenges that researchers have to face, either for the development of an accepted gluten vehicle and placebo or for identifying NCGS cases on the basis of DBPC gluten challenges.

Keywords: celiac disease; wheat; gluten; non-celiac gluten-sensitivity; diagnosis

---

1. Introduction

Wheat is one of the most consumed cereals in western countries [1], but some wheat components trigger the diseases encompassed under the term gluten-related disorders [2]. These diseases principally include celiac disease, wheat allergy, and the new clinical entity non-celiac gluten-sensitivity (NCGS) [3,4]. The diagnosis of the first two conditions can be supported by using blood-based diagnostic tests, whereas there is a lack of reliable biomarkers for the diagnosis of NCGS [4]. Thus, experts of gluten-related disorders have proposed that single- or double-blind placebo-controlled (DBPC) gluten challenges should be carried out to establish the diagnosis of NCGS, either for clinical practice (single-blind) or research purposes (double-blind) [5]. The challenges have to be carried out using cooked gluten, and the gluten vehicle and placebo must be indistinguishable from each other [5]. However, no study has proposed a gluten vehicle and placebo that meet the characteristics given by the experts. Consequently, there is a huge heterogeneity in the characteristics of the gluten vehicles and placebo used for carrying out DBPC gluten challenges for NCGS assessment [6,7]. This complicates comparisons among studies [8] and highlights the need of standardized gluten vehicle and placebo accepted by the scientific and clinical communities. In this narrative review, we present advances on the design of both gluten vehicle and placebo used for NCGS assessment.

2. DBPC Gluten Challenges

There are some variables that should be taken into account when interpreting the outcomes of DBPC gluten challenges (Figure 1). The challenge, as stated in The Salerno experts' criteria, involves two stages: (1) assessing the clinical response to a gluten-free diet (GFD) and (2) assessing the effect of reintroducing gluten after a period of treatment with the GFD [5]. In each stage, the patients use a self-administered instrument, which is called Gastrointestinal Symptom Rating Scale (GSRS). This instrument evaluates in a scale from 1 (mild) to 10 (severe) the gastrointestinal and extra-intestinal manifestations associated with NCGS [5]. In stage 1 (response to a gluten-free diet), a reduction >30% of the symptomatic baseline score for one to three main symptoms or at least one symptom with no worsening of the others is needed to pass to the second stage. In stage 2 (DBPC gluten challenge with crossover), data about the symptoms during the gluten and placebo challenge are collected. Differences in the scores of the GSRS of at least 30% are required to discriminate a positive response from a negative result [6]. However, some points in this diagnostic approach have not been carefully considered by some researchers. As shown in Table 1, the time periods reported for carrying out DBPC gluten-challenges vary from 1 day to 6 months, although challenges shorter than one week might not detect fluctuating symptoms [9].

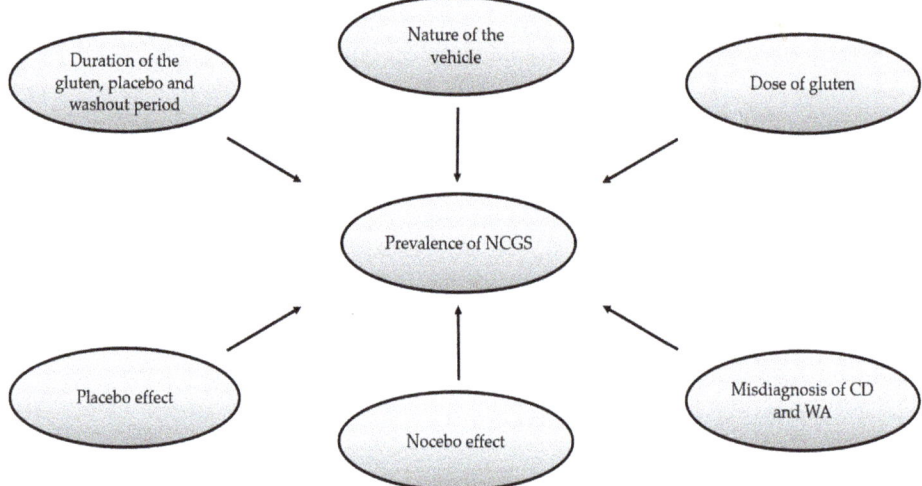

Figure 1. Factors that influence non-celiac gluten sensitivity (NCGS) assessment using double-blind placebo-controlled (DBPC) gluten challenges. CD: celiac disease, WA: wheat allergy.

Regarding the doses of gluten, these vary from 2 g/day to 52 g/day [10,11], and this variation could impact the symptomatic outcomes. In fact, Zanini et al. [12] estimated an NCGS prevalence rate of 34% using a vehicle containing 7.9 g of gluten and a 10-day gluten challenge, but others estimated half of that prevalence using a vehicle containing 4.7 to 5.6 g of gluten in a 7-day gluten challenge [7,8,13]. Besides the dose of gluten utilized for the challenges and the time of gluten exposure, another factor that deserves attention is the washout period. Some authors have recommended washout periods for more than one week when carrying out DBPC gluten challenges. This is to ensure specificity and to prevent fluctuating symptoms [8]. Overall, there is a huge heterogeneity regarding the parameters of time of gluten exposure, dose of gluten, and washout period utilized for carrying out the DBPC gluten challenge for NCGS assessment, either in clinical or research settings (Table 1).

Table 1. Studies reporting DBPC gluten challenge results for NCGS assessment. GSRS-IBS: Gastrointestinal Symptom Rating Scale-Irritable bowel syndrome

Study/Design	No. Patients	Presentation/Dose of Gluten	Placebo Vehicle	Gluten Challenge	Washout Period	Outcomes
Biesiekierski et al., 2011—DBPCT [14]	34	Bread and muffin, 16 g/day	Bread and muffin	6 weeks		13 patients (68%) in the gluten group reported symptoms that were not adequately controlled, but 6 patients (40%) in the placebo group reported the symptoms.
Biesiekierski et al., 2013—DBPCT with cross-over [10]	37	Diet High: 16 g/day Low: 2 g/day	16 g whey protein	1 week	Up to 2 weeks	The symptoms improved in all the participants (n = 37) during a low-FODMAP diet, although adverse reactions to gluten were reported by 8% (n = 3) of the patients.
Peters et al., 2014—DBPCT with cross-over [15]	22	Diet 16 g/day	16 g whey protein or placebo	3 days	At least 3 days	Gluten ingestion was associated with a high overall symptoms-based score of depression (63%; n = 14) in comparison to the ingestion of placebo (36%; n = 8).
Shahbazkhani et al., 2015—DBPCT [16]	72	Gluten meal powder, 52 g/day	Gluten-free meal powder (rice flour, corn starch, and glucose)	6 weeks	-	The symptoms were better controlled in the placebo group than in the group that received gluten (83.8%; n = 31 and 25.7%; n = 9, respectively).
Di Sabatino et al., 2015—DBPCT with cross-over [13]	61	Gastrosoluble capsules, 4.375 g/day	Gastrosoluble capsules, 4.375 g/day rice starch	1 week	1 week	Gluten intake significantly increased the overall symptoms in comparison to the placebo group. However, only three patients were defined as NCGS subjects (5%).
Zanini et al., 2015—DBPCT with cross-over [12]	35	Flour, 7.9 g/day	Flour, 7.67 starch, 0.68 g lactose, 0.01 g fructans	10 days	2 weeks	12 (34%) out of 35 participants were classified as NCGS patients, but 17 (49%) of the participants reported symptoms during the placebo challenge.
Elli et al., 2016 DBPCT with cross-over [7]	98	Gastrosoluble capsules, 5.6 g/day	Gastrosoluble capsules, 5.6 g/day rice starch	1 week	1 week	28 out of 98 patients reported symptomatic relapse during gluten ingestion. However, only 14% of those that reacted to gluten ingestion did not respond to the placebo challenge.
Picarelli et al., 2016-DBPCT with cross-over [17]	26	Crosssaint, 10 g/day	Gluten-free croissant	1 day	-	Eight (61.5%) out of 13 NCGS patients reported a high overall score of symptoms during the gluten challenge. However, in a second group, 6 (46.2%) out of 13 NCGS patients reported symptomatic relapse during the placebo challenge.
Rosinach et al., 2016 [18]-DBPCT	18	Sachets, 16.2 g/day	Gluten-free sachets	6 months	-	Ten (91%) out of 11 participants reported adverse reactions after gluten ingestion. In a second group, only two (28.5%) out of seven participants reported symptomatic relapse after placebo ingestion.
Skodje et al., 2018 [19]—DBPCT with cross-over	59	Muesli bar, 5.7 g/day	2.1 g fructan/placebo muesli bar	1 week	At least 7 days	Symptomatic response in the placebo group (37.28%) was higher than in the group that received gluten (22.03%). The overall GSRS-IBS score was higher in the fructan group (44%) than in the group that received gluten (22%). However, no significant difference in the overall GSRS-IBS score between the fructan group (44%) and the placebo group (37%) was found.
Dale et al., 2018 [20]—DBPCT with cross-over	20	Muffin, 11 g/day	Gluten-free muffin	4 days	3 days	Only 4 out of 20 patients were diagnosed with NCGS (20%). Patients that did not meet the criteria for NCGS (80%) reported more severe symptoms with placebo than with gluten.
Francavilla et al., 2018 [21]—DBPCT with cross-over	28	Sachets, 10 g/day	Gluten-free starch sachets	2 weeks	1 week	Eleven (39.3%) out of 28 patients were classified as NCGS cases.

Additionally, researchers and clinicians should take into account the placebo and nocebo effects, as the manifestations of symptoms during the gluten and placebo challenge may be similar [22]. In fact, the nocebo effect could be as high as 40% in DBPC studies [8]. On the side of the positive conditioning, the studies by Dale et al. [20] and by Skodje et al. [19] reported higher manifestations of symptoms during the placebo challenge (up to 37%) than during the gluten challenge (22%). In this context, it has been proposed that increasing the ratio placebo challenges/gluten challenges to 2:1 can be an effective strategy to minimize false-positive cases [23].

According to the Salerno experts, the characteristics of the gluten vehicle and placebo utilized for carrying out the DBPC gluten challenge should be as follows: "The gluten and placebo preparations must be undistinguishable in look, texture and taste, and balanced in fibers, carbohydrate, fat and possible protein" [5]. This implies a big challenge for food science technologists mainly due to the viscoelastic properties of gluten, which strongly impact on the texture and appearance of gluten-containing products. In fact, the technological and sensory properties provided by gluten are difficult to mimic in gluten-free products [24], and no study conducted to rule in or rule out NCGS has reported the use of a gluten vehicle and placebo that meet the characteristics given by the Salerno experts (Table 2). Thus, to identify NCGS cases, the design and the widespread use of a gluten vehicle and placebo that meet the characteristics proposed by the experts or of other gluten vehicle and placebo accepted by scientists and clinicians seem urgent.

Table 2. Characteristics of the gluten vehicle and placebo proposed by the Salerno experts and the characteristics proposed by others.

Study	Presentation	Gluten GV	Gluten PV	ATIs GV	ATIs PV	FODMAP GV	FODMAP PV	Protein GV PV	Fat GV PV	HC GV PV
Salerno experts Catassi et al., 2015 [5]	It can be a muesli bar, bread, muffin or may differ between children and adults.	8 g/day	Free	0.3 g/8 g gluten	Free	Free	Free	Possible balanced	Balanced	Balanced
Elli et al., 2016 [7]	Gastrosoluble capsules	5.6 g/day	Free	NR	NR	NR	Low-FODMAP	NR	NR	NR
Rosinach et al., 2016 [18]	Sachets	16.2 g/day	Free	NR	NR	Free	Free	Not balanced	Not balanced	Not balanced
Skyje et al., 2018 [19]	Muesli bar	5.7 g/day	Free	Free	Free	Free	Free	Possible balanced	Balanced	Balanced
Dale et al., 2018 [20]	Muffin	11 g/day	Free	NR	NR	Low-FODMAP	Low-FODMAP	Possible balanced	Balanced	Balanced
Francavilla et al., 2018 [21]	Sachets	10 g/day	Free	0.4g	Free	Free	Free	Possible balanced	Balanced	Balanced

Acronyms used: GV: gluten vehicle, PV: placebo vehicle, ATIs: amylase and trypsin inhibitors, FODMAP: fermentable oligo-, di-, monosaccharides, and polyols, HC: Carbohydrates, NR: not reported.

3. Current State of NCGS

NCGS is defined as "a syndrome characterized by intestinal and extra-intestinal symptoms related to the ingestion of gluten-containing food, in subjects that are not affected by either celiac disease or wheat allergy" [5]. Although the real prevalence of NCGS remains unknown, current data suggest that it ranges from 0.6% to 6% in the general population [25–29]. One of the major challenges in the diagnosis of NCGS is the identification of the components that trigger the manifestations reported [9,30]. This is an area that remains poorly understood and has been the object of extensive research. Certainly, there are different components that may cause adverse reactions in NCGS patients, such as gluten, FODMAPs (fermentable oligo-, di-, monosaccharides, and polyols) and ATIs (amylase and trypsin inhibitors) [31]. According to some authors, NCGS individuals are sensitive to one or another, if not all, of these wheat components [32,33]. Furthermore, there is a huge spectrum of both gastrointestinal and extraintestinal manifestations [34]. In line with this, it is suggested that the pathogenesis of NCGS should be drawn taking into account the collective effect of the wheat components [35]. In this case, the gluten vehicle and placebo utilized for carrying out DBPC gluten challenges for identifying NCGS cases should include standardized amounts of the main suspected triggers of the condition.

4. Characteristics of the Gluten Vehicle and Placebo for Carrying out DBPC Gluten Challenges

According to experts, the gluten vehicle for carrying out DBPC gluten challenges should contain cooked and homogeneously distributed gluten (8 g per dose) and the pro-inflammatory factor ATIs (0.3 g/8 g of gluten) and be FODMAPs-free [5]. The use of gelatin capsules is discouraged, and this has motivated the search for the best-suited gluten vehicle. However, changes in the content of gluten, ATIs, and FODMAPs modify the food matrix structure altering the sensory characteristics of the food. From a commercial point of view, the more similar the gluten-free product is to its gluten-containing counterpart the better it is, but for the purpose of a gluten vehicle and placebo indistinguishable from each other for carrying out DBPC gluten challenges, this is not the rule. The development of a gluten vehicle could start from a gluten-free base formulation, trying to preserve the characteristics when gluten is added. To exclude variations of some of the sensory characteristics, drying and milling of the gluten vehicle and placebo until a flour-like material is obtained could be helpful [36]. Certainly, the challenge for developing an appropriate vehicle for gluten administration and its respective placebo is to maintain them indistinguishable from each other, while keeping the placebo in gluten-, ATIs-, and FODMAPs-free conditions.

4.1. Sensory and Technological Characteristics Given by Gluten to Baked Food Products

Gluten represents 80–85% of the total protein from wheat [37] and includes two main subgroups of proteins: gliadin (alcohol-soluble fraction) and glutenins (weak acid-soluble fraction) [38]. These two proteins are responsible for many technological properties of baked food products. For instance, hydrated gliadins contribute mainly to the viscosity and extensibility of the dough, and hydrated glutenins confer cohesive and elastic properties, which are responsible for dough strength and elasticity [39]. Furthermore, interactions between both gliadins and glutenins increase dough viscosity and, at the same time, decrease the high level of elasticity conferred by glutenins. This balance between gliadins and glutenins are determinant for dough rheology [40] and, consequently, some additives are used in the preparation of most gluten-free baked goods to mimic the technological characteristics given by gluten. Thus, as shown in Table 1, some authors evaluate the sensory and/or technological characteristics of a designed gluten-free product and compare it with the same product without gluten additives instead of comparing it with the gluten-containing product, which is the one being surrogated. Others have reported sensory evaluations of both gluten vehicle and placebo to ensure that they were indistinguishable from each other (Table 1). However, the specific formulations and methods of preparation have not been reported, making it difficult to replicate the results obtained by different research groups.

4.2. Sensory and Technological Characteristics Given by FODMAPs to Baked Food Products

FODMAPs are a group of components encompassing oligosaccharides (fructo-oligosaccharides), disaccharides (lactose), monosaccharides (fructose), and polyols (sorbitol, mannitol, maltitol, xylitol, polydextrose, and isomalt). The consumption of FODMAPs may trigger adverse reactions in susceptible individuals [41]. The mechanisms underlying the symptoms triggered by FODMAPs can be categorized as follows: (1) poor absorption of fructose, polyols, and lactose in the small intestine, (2) activation of an osmotic effect due to the small size of FODMAPs and stimulation of mechanoreceptors that increase luminal water content, and (3) a high rate of FODMAPs fermentation by bacteria [42,43]. Certainly, FODMAPs are part of the suspected dietary components that can trigger the gastrointestinal symptoms seen in NCGS cases [10]. Therefore, the Salerno experts' criteria established that the vehicles used for carrying out DBPC gluten challenges have to be FODMAPs-free, but just a few studies have reported the use of a FODMAPs-free placebo (Table 1). Understanding the role of FODMAPs in the food matrix of baked food products is important for designing a gluten vehicle and placebo with potential to be indistinguishable from each other.

The disaccharide sucrose (glucose plus fructose) can interact with other food ingredients and modify the sensory and physical properties of food products, such as sweetness, flavor, color formation, and texture [44]. Because sucrose provides more sweetness than other mono- and di-saccharides, such as maltose and glucose, its presence can increase the sweet flavor in many cereal-based products [45]. Furthermore, sucrose is important for the aeration of baked products, a process that increases the volumetric aeration rate and decreases the bubble size [46]. On the other hand, oligosaccharides (saccharides containing 3–10 sugar moieties) confer low-intensity sweetness to foods [47] but provide increased viscosity, improving the body and mouthfeel of food products [48]. In addition, oligosaccharides and other sugars are important for browning intensity throughout Maillard reactions and provide a high moisture-retaining capacity, preventing excessive drying [48]. For the purposes of DBPC gluten challenges for NCGS assessment, both gluten vehicle and placebo have to be FODMAPs-free. Thus, the technological and sensory characteristics given by FODMAPs to baked foods would not be of relevance in the design of a gluten vehicle and placebo, but researchers should take into account that the absence of both FODMAPs and gluten in a food matrix makes more feasible the design of a gluten vehicle and a placebo different from a bakery product.

4.3. Sensory and Technological Characteristics Given by ATIs to Baked Food Products

ATIs are a group of low-molecular-weight proteins (~15 kDa) that have amylase and trypsin inhibitory properties and represent ~4% of the total protein content in wheat flour [33,49]. They have been proposed as the potential triggers of the manifestations seen in NCGS cases [50]. ATIs from wheat, rye, and barley, but not from other plant species, can activate the innate immune system throughout their interaction with toll-like receptor 4, giving rise to TLR4-MD2-CD14 complexes and promoting the release of proinflammatory cytokines by myeloid cells [51,52]. Amylases are used mainly in fermented bakery products. These enzymes degrade the flour starch into dextrins allowing dough fermentation by yeasts. This process improves the volume of fermented breads and crumb texture [53]. Furthermore, amylases catalysis increases the content of fermentable and reducing sugars in flour, promoting the formation of Maillard reactions, which intensify bread flavor and crust color [54]. Regarding trypsin, it reduces the mixing time of flour dough and improves some sensory properties of bakery products, such as texture, flavor, and crust color of a bread loaf [55,56]. Thus, the sensory and technological characteristics given by ATIs to baked foods other than fermented bread seems not to be as relevant as those given by gluten and FODMAPs. However, it remains to be evaluated in detail whether the presence or absence of 0.3 g of ATIs/8 g of gluten involves significant changes of the technological and sensory characteristics of baked food products.

5. Perspectives

Although anti-gliadin IgG [57,58] and anti-nucleus antibodies seem to be associated with NCGS [58,59], there is still a lack of highly sensitive and specific serological biomarkers for NCGS, and the most accepted diagnostic algorithm for this clinical entity includes DBPC gluten challenges as the cornerstone. There are some non-standardized points in such an approach, which complicate fair comparisons among studies focused on the identification of NCGS. The most notable of these points is the lack of a gluten vehicle and a placebo that meet the characteristics given by the Salerno experts. The gluten vehicle and placebo must be indistinguishable from each other. In this context, sensory evaluations can be considered mandatory if the research purpose is the design of a gluten vehicle and a placebo for carrying out DBPC gluten challenges for NCGS assessment. Furthermore, the full recipe and method of preparation of the gluten vehicle and placebo should be clearly stated in order to promote the replication of the results and the acceptance of the proposed methodology by the scientific and clinical communities.

Biomarkers at intestinal level have been proposed to aid in the diagnosis of NCGS. On one hand, histological evaluations suggest that eosinophils (increased number) could be an intestinal biomarker for NCGS [60,61], while others have proposed the evaluation of mast cells, T helper, and intraepithelial lymphocytes [62]. On the other hand, expression analyses of immune molecules such as tissue transglutaminase 2, interferon gamma, toll-like receptor 2, and myeloid differentiation factor 88 are less promising as a diagnostic tool [63], although these analyses are of relevance to elucidate the pathogenic mechanisms that underlie NCGS [64]. The main limitation of these tests is that they include an invasive procedure. The tests are reliable in patients on a gluten-containing diet, but standardized gluten challenges should be carried out for patients already following a gluten-free diet. For instance, a three-day gluten challenge with cooked and homogeneously distributed gluten can trigger T cell immunity to gluten without causing significant architectural disruption to the small intestinal mucosa in celiac disease cases, but they do not trigger T cell immunity to gluten in NCGS individuals [65,66]. Because of the invasive nature of intestinal biomarkers evaluation, biopsy-proven NCGS assessment should only be considered in well-established symptomatic cases of gluten intake. These cases should be identified on the basis of DBPC gluten challenges, carried out using a gluten vehicle and a placebo indistinguishable from each other. As mentioned before, such gluten vehicle and placebo are still to be developed, but we believe that the conditions exist for a close collaboration between cereal technologists and clinical researchers for developing accepted gluten vehicle and placebo for NCGS diagnosis purposes.

Author Contributions: Conceptualization, O.G.F.-S., N.O., and F.C.-C.; Investigation, O.G.F.-S., N.O., and F.C.-C.; Original Draft Preparation O.G.F.-S., N.O., and F.C.-C.; Writing—Review & Editing, O.G.F.-S., N.O., and F.C.-C.

Funding: This research received no external funding.

Conflicts of Interest: The authors declare no conflict of interest.

References

1. Dale, H.F.; Biesiekierski, J.R.; Lied, G.A. Non-coeliac gluten sensitivity and the spectrum of gluten-related disorders: An updated overview. *Nutr. Res. Rev.* **2018**, *16*, 1–10. [CrossRef]
2. Leonard, M.M.; Vasagar, B. US perspective on gluten-related diseases. *Clin. Exp. Gastroenterol.* **2014**, *7*, 25.
3. Ludvigsson, J.F.; Leffler, D.A.; Bai, J.C.; Biagi, F.; Fasano, A.; Green, P.H.; Hadjivassiliou, M.; Kaukinen, K.; Kelly, C.P.; Leonard, J.N.; et al. The Oslo definitions for coeliac disease and related terms. *Gut* **2013**, *62*, 43–52. [CrossRef]
4. Ontiveros, N.; Hardy, M.; Cabrera-Chavez, F. Assessing of celiac disease and nonceliac gluten sensitivity. *Gastroenterol. Res. Pract.* **2015**, *2015*, 723954. [CrossRef]
5. Catassi, C.; Elli, L.; Bonaz, B.; Bouma, G.; Carroccio, A.; Castillejo, G.; Cellier, C.; Cristofori, F.; de Magistris, L.; Dolinsek, J. Diagnosis of non-celiac gluten sensitivity (NCGS): The Salerno experts' criteria. *Nutrients* **2015**, *7*, 4966–4977. [CrossRef]
6. Bonciolini, V.; Bianchi, B.; Del Bianco, E.; Verdelli, A.; Caproni, M. Cutaneous manifestations of non-celiac gluten sensitivity: Clinical histological and immunopathological features. *Nutrients* **2015**, *7*, 7798–7805. [CrossRef]
7. Elli, L.; Tomba, C.; Branchi, F.; Roncoroni, L.; Lombardo, V.; Bardella, M.T.; Ferretti, F.; Conte, D.; Valiante, F.; Fini, L. Evidence for the presence of non-celiac gluten sensitivity in patients with functional gastrointestinal symptoms: Results from a multicenter randomized double-blind placebo-controlled gluten challenge. *Nutrients* **2016**, *8*, 84. [CrossRef]
8. Molina-Infante, J.; Carroccio, A. Suspected nonceliac gluten sensitivity confirmed in few patients after gluten challenge in double-blind, placebo-controlled trials. *Clin. Gastroenterol. Hepatol.* **2017**, *15*, 339–348. [CrossRef]
9. Catassi, C.; Alaedini, A.; Bojarski, C.; Bonaz, B.; Bouma, G.; Carroccio, A.; Castillejo, G.; De Magistris, L.; Dieterich, W.; Di Liberto, D. The overlapping area of non-celiac gluten sensitivity (NCGS) and wheat-sensitive irritable bowel syndrome (IBS): An update. *Nutrients* **2017**, *9*, 1268. [CrossRef]
10. Biesiekierski, J.R.; Peters, S.L.; Newnham, E.D.; Rosella, O.; Muir, J.G.; Gibson, P.R. No effects of gluten in patients with self-reported non-celiac gluten sensitivity after dietary reduction of fermentable, poorly absorbed, short-chain carbohydrates. *Gastroenterology* **2013**, *145*. [CrossRef]

11. Zanwar, V.G.; Pawar, S.V.; Gambhire, P.A.; Jain, S.S.; Surude, R.G.; Shah, V.B.; Contractor, Q.Q.; Rathi, P.M. Symptomatic improvement with gluten restriction in irritable bowel syndrome: A prospective, randomized, double blinded placebo controlled trial. *Intest. Res.* **2016**, *14*, 343–350. [CrossRef]
12. Zanini, B.; Baschè, R.; Ferraresi, A.; Ricci, C.; Lanzarotto, F.; Marullo, M.; Villanacci, V.; Hidalgo, A.; Lanzini, A. Randomised clinical study: Gluten challenge induces symptom recurrence in only a minority of patients who meet clinical criteria for non-coeliac gluten sensitivity. *Aliment. Pharmacol. Ther.* **2015**, *42*, 968–976. [CrossRef]
13. Di Sabatino, A.; Volta, U.; Salvatore, C.; Biancheri, P.; Caio, G.; De Giorgio, R.; Di Stefano, M.; Corazza, G.R. Small amounts of gluten in subjects with suspected nonceliac gluten sensitivity: A randomized, double-blind, placebo-controlled, cross-over trial. *Clin. Gastroenterol. Hepatol.* **2015**, *13*, 1604–1612. [CrossRef]
14. Biesiekierski, J.R.; Newnham, E.D.; Irving, P.M.; Barrett, J.S.; Haines, M.; Doecke, J.D.; Shepherd, S.J.; Muir, J.G.; Gibson, P.R. Gluten causes gastrointestinal symptoms in subjects without celiac disease: A double-blind randomized placebo-controlled trial. *Am. J. Gastroenterol.* **2011**, *106*, 508. [CrossRef]
15. Peters, S.; Biesiekierski, J.; Yelland, G.; Muir, J.; Gibson, P. Randomised clinical trial: Gluten may cause depression in subjects with non-coeliac gluten sensitivity–an exploratory clinical study. *Aliment. Pharmacol. Ther.* **2014**, *39*, 1104–1112. [CrossRef]
16. Shahbazkhani, B.; Sadeghi, A.; Malekzadeh, R.; Khatavi, F.; Etemadi, M.; Kalantri, E.; Rostami-Nejad, M.; Rostami, K. Non-celiac gluten sensitivity has narrowed the spectrum of irritable bowel syndrome: A double-blind randomized placebo-controlled trial. *Nutrients* **2015**, *7*, 4542–4554. [CrossRef]
17. Picarelli, A.; Borghini, R.; Di Tola, M.; Marino, M.; Urciuoli, C.; Isonne, C.; Puzzono, M.; Porowska, B.; Rumi, G.; Lonardi, S. Intestinal, systemic, and oral gluten-related alterations in patients with nonceliac gluten sensitivity. *J. Clin. Gastroenterol.* **2016**, *50*, 849–858. [CrossRef]
18. Rosinach, M.; Fernández-Bañares, F.; Carrasco, A.; Ibarra, M.; Temiño, R.; Salas, A.; Esteve, M. Double-Blind randomized clinical trial: Gluten versus placebo rechallenge in patients with lymphocytic enteritis and suspected celiac disease. *PLoS ONE* **2016**, *11*, e0157879. [CrossRef]
19. Skodje, G.I.; Sarna, V.K.; Minelle, I.H.; Rolfsen, K.L.; Muir, J.G.; Gibson, P.R.; Veierød, M.B.; Henriksen, C.; Lundin, K.E. Fructan, rather than gluten, induces symptoms in patients with self-reported non-celiac gluten sensitivity. *Gastroenterology* **2018**, *154*, 529–539. [CrossRef]
20. Dale, H.; Hatlebakk, J.; Hovdenak, N.; Ystad, S.; Lied, G. The effect of a controlled gluten challenge in a group of patients with suspected non-coeliac gluten sensitivity: A randomized, double-blind placebo-controlled challenge. *Neurogastroenterol. Motil.* **2018**. [CrossRef]
21. Francavilla, R.; Cristofori, F.; Verzillo, L.; Gentile, A.; Castellaneta, S.; Polloni, C.; Giorgio, V.; Verduci, E.; D'Angelo, E.; Dellatte, S. Randomized double-blind placebo-controlled crossover trial for the diagnosis of non-celiac gluten sensitivity in children. *Am. J. Gastroenterol.* **2018**, *113*, 421. [CrossRef]
22. Lionetti, E.; Pulvirenti, A.; Vallorani, M.; Catassi, G.; Verma, A.K.; Gatti, S.; Catassi, C. Re-challenge studies in non-celiac gluten sensitivity: A systematic review and meta-analysis. *Front. Phys.* **2017**, *8*, 621. [CrossRef]
23. Reese, I.; Schäfer, C.; Kleine-Tebbe, J.; Ahrens, B.; Bachmann, O.; Ballmer-Weber, B.; Beyer, K.; Bischoff, S.C.; Blümchen, K.; Dölle, S. Non-celiac gluten/wheat sensitivity (NCGS)—a currently undefined disorder without validated diagnostic criteria and of unknown prevalence. *Allergo J. Int.* **2018**, *27*, 1–5. [CrossRef]
24. Hosseini, S.M.; Soltanizadeh, N.; Mirmoghtadaee, P.; Banavand, P.; Mirmoghtadaie, L.; Shojaee-Aliabadi, S. Gluten-free products in celiac disease: Nutritional and technological challenges and solutions. *J. Res. Med. Sci. Off. J. Isfahan Univ. Med. Sci.* **2018**, *23*, 109.
25. Aziz, I. *The Global Phenomenon of Self-Reported Wheat Sensitivity*; Nature Publishing Group: London, UK, 2018.
26. Ontiveros, N.; López-Gallardo, J.A.; Vergara-Jiménez, M.J.; Cabrera-Chávez, F. Self-reported prevalence of symptomatic adverse reactions to gluten and adherence to gluten-free diet in an adult Mexican population. *Nutrients* **2015**, *7*, 6000–6015. [CrossRef]
27. Cabrera-Chávez, F.; Granda-Restrepo, D.M.; Arámburo-Gálvez, J.G.; Franco-Aguilar, A.; Magaña-Ordorica, D.; Vergara-Jiménez, M.d.J.; Ontiveros, N. Self-reported prevalence of gluten-related disorders and adherence to gluten-free diet in Colombian adult population. *Gastroenterol. Res. Pract.* **2016**, *2016*, 4704309. [CrossRef]
28. Cabrera-Chávez, F.; Dezar, G.; Islas-Zamorano, A.; Espinoza-Alderete, J.; Vergara-Jiménez, M.; Magaña-Ordorica, D.; Ontiveros, N. Prevalence of self-reported gluten sensitivity and adherence to a gluten-free diet in argentinian adult population. *Nutrients* **2017**, *9*, 81. [CrossRef]

29. Ontiveros, N.; Rodríguez-Bellegarrigue, C.; Galicia-Rodríguez, G.; Vergara-Jiménez, M.; Zepeda-Gómez, E.; Arámburo-Galvez, J.; Gracia-Valenzuela, M.; Cabrera-Chávez, F. Prevalence of self-reported gluten-related disorders and adherence to a gluten-free diet in Salvadoran adult population. *Int. J. Environ. Res. Public Health* **2018**, *15*, 786. [CrossRef]
30. Krigel, A.; Lebwohl, B. Nonceliac gluten sensitivity. *Adv. Nutr.* **2016**, *7*, 1105–1110. [CrossRef]
31. Collyer, E.M.; Kaplan, B.S. Nonceliac gluten sensitivity: An approach to diagnosis and management. *Curr. Opin. Pediatr.* **2016**, *28*, 638–643. [CrossRef]
32. Dieterich, W.; Schuppan, D.; Schink, M.; Schwappacher, R.; Wirtz, S.; Agaimy, A.; Neurath, M.F.; Zopf, Y. Influence of low FODMAP and gluten-free diets on disease activity and intestinal microbiota in patients with non-celiac gluten sensitivity. *Clin. Nutr.* **2018**, *10*, 1708. [CrossRef] [PubMed]
33. Reig-Otero, Y.; Manes, J.; Manyes, L. Amylase–Trypsin Inhibitors in Wheat and Other Cereals as Potential Activators of the Effects of Nonceliac Gluten Sensitivity. *J. Med. Food* **2018**, *21*, 207–214. [CrossRef] [PubMed]
34. Igbinedion, S.O.; Ansari, J.; Vasikaran, A.; Gavins, F.N.; Jordan, P.; Boktor, M.; Alexander, J.S. Non-celiac gluten sensitivity: All wheat attack is not celiac. *World J. Gastroenterol.* **2017**, *23*, 7201. [CrossRef] [PubMed]
35. Volta, U.; De Giorgio, R.; Caio, G.; Uhde, M.; Manfredini, R.; Alaedini, A. Nonceliac Wheat Sensitivity: An Immune-Mediated Condition with Systemic Manifestations. *Gastroenterol. Clin.* **2018**, *48*, 165–182. [CrossRef] [PubMed]
36. Goel, G.; King, T.; Daveson, A.J.; Andrews, J.M.; Krishnarajah, J.; Krause, R.; Brown, G.J.; Fogel, R.; Barish, C.F.; Epstein, R. Epitope-specific immunotherapy targeting CD4-positive T cells in coeliac disease: Two randomised, double-blind, placebo-controlled phase 1 studies. *Lancet Gastroenterol. Hepatol.* **2017**, *2*, 479–493. [CrossRef]
37. Anjum, F.M.; Khan, M.R.; Din, A.; Saeed, M.; Pasha, I.; Arshad, M.U. Wheat gluten: High molecular weight glutenin subunits—structure, genetics, and relation to dough elasticity. *J. Food Sci.* **2007**, *72*, R56–R63. [CrossRef]
38. Biesiekierski, J.R. What is gluten? *J. Gastroenterol. Hepatol.* **2017**, *32*, 78–81. [CrossRef]
39. Wieser, H. Chemistry of gluten proteins. *Food Microbiol.* **2007**, *24*, 115–119. [CrossRef]
40. Ortolan, F.; Steel, C.J. Protein characteristics that affect the quality of vital wheat gluten to be used in baking: A review. *Compr. Rev. Food Sci. Food Saf.* **2017**, *16*, 369–381.
41. Catassi, G.; Lionetti, E.; Gatti, S.; Catassi, C. The low FODMAP diet: Many question marks for a catchy acronym. *Nutrients* **2017**, *9*, 292. [CrossRef]
42. Hill, P.; Muir, J.G.; Gibson, P.R. Controversies and recent developments of the low-FODMAP diet. *Gastroenterol. Hepatol.* **2017**, *13*, 36.
43. Zannini, E.; Arendt, E.K. Low FODMAPs and gluten-free foods for irritable bowel syndrome treatment: Lights and shadows. *Food Res. Int.* **2018**, *110*, 33–41. [CrossRef]
44. Goldfein, K.R.; Slavin, J.L. Why sugar is added to food: Food science 101. *Compr. Rev. Food Sci. Food Saf.* **2015**, *14*, 644–656. [CrossRef]
45. Pareyt, B.; Delcour, J.A. The role of wheat flour constituents, sugar, and fat in low moisture cereal based products: A review on sugar-snap cookies. *Crit. Rev. Food Sci. Nutr.* **2008**, *48*, 824–839. [CrossRef]
46. Trinh, L.; Lowe, T.; Campbell, G.M.; Withers, P.; Martin, P. Effect of sugar on bread dough aeration during mixing. *J. Food Eng.* **2015**, *150*, 9–18. [CrossRef]
47. Meyer, T.S.M.; Miguel, Â.S.M.; Fernández, D.E.R.; Ortiz, G.M.D. Biotechnological production of oligosaccharides-applications in the food industry. In *Food Production and Industry*; Eissa, A.A., Ed.; Intech Open: Rijeka, Croatia, 2015.
48. Mussatto, S.I.; Mancilha, I.M. Non-digestible oligosaccharides: A review. *Carbohydr. Polym.* **2007**, *68*, 587–597. [CrossRef]
49. Schuppan, D.; Pickert, G.; Ashfaq-Khan, M.; Zevallos, V. Non-celiac wheat sensitivity: Differential diagnosis, triggers and implications. *Best Pract. Res. Clin. Gastroenterol.* **2015**, *29*, 469–476. [CrossRef]
50. Schuppan, D.; Zevallos, V. Wheat amylase trypsin inhibitors as nutritional activators of innate immunity. *Dig. Dis.* **2015**, *33*, 260–263. [CrossRef]
51. Zevallos, V.F.; Raker, V.; Tenzer, S.; Jimenez-Calvente, C.; Ashfaq-Khan, M.; Rüssel, N.; Pickert, G.; Schild, H.; Steinbrink, K.; Schuppan, D. Nutritional wheat amylase-trypsin inhibitors promote intestinal inflammation via activation of myeloid cells. *Gastroenterology* **2017**, *152*, 1100–1113. [CrossRef]

52. Junker, Y.; Zeissig, S.; Kim, S.-J.; Barisani, D.; Wieser, H.; Leffler, D.A.; Zevallos, V.; Libermann, T.A.; Dillon, S.; Freitag, T.L. Wheat amylase trypsin inhibitors drive intestinal inflammation via activation of toll-like receptor 4. *J. Exp. Med.* **2012**, *209*, 2395–2408. [CrossRef]
53. Saini, R.; Saini, H.S.; Dahiya, A. Amylases: Characteristics and industrial applications. *J. Pharmacogn. Phytochem.* **2017**, *6*, 1865–1871.
54. Goesaert, H.; Slade, L.; Levine, H.; Delcour, J.A. Amylases and bread firming–an integrated view. *J. Cereal Sci.* **2009**, *50*, 345–352. [CrossRef]
55. Tavano, O.L. Protein hydrolysis using proteases: An important tool for food biotechnology. *J. Mol. Catal. B Enzym.* **2013**, *90*, 1–11. [CrossRef]
56. Singh, R.; Singh, A.; Sachan, S. Enzymes Used in the Food Industry: Friends or Foes. In *Enzymes in Food Biotechnology*, 1st ed.; Kuddus, M., Ed.; Elsevier: Amsterdam, The Netherlands, 2019; pp. 827–843.
57. Volta, U.; Tovoli, F.; Cicola, R.; Parisi, C.; Fabbri, A.; Piscaglia, M.; Fiorini, E.; Caio, G. Serological tests in gluten sensitivity (nonceliac gluten intolerance). *J. Clin. Gastroenterol.* **2012**, *46*, 680–685. [CrossRef]
58. Losurdo, G.; Principi, M.; Iannone, A.; Giangaspero, A.; Piscitelli, D.; Ierardi, E.; Di Leo, A.; Barone, M. Predictivity of autoimmune stigmata for gluten sensitivity in subjects with microscopic enteritis: A retrospective study. *Nutrients* **2018**, *10*, 2001. [CrossRef]
59. Carroccio, A.; D'Alcamo, A.; Cavataio, F.; Soresi, M.; Seidita, A.; Sciumè, C.; Geraci, G.; Iacono, G.; Mansueto, P. High proportions of people with nonceliac wheat sensitivity have autoimmune disease or antinuclear antibodies. *Gastroenterology* **2015**, *149*, 596–603. [CrossRef]
60. Carroccio, A.; Giannone, G.; Mansueto, P.; Soresi, M.; La Blasca, F.; Fayer, F.; Iacobucci, R.; Porcasi, R.; Catalano, T.; Geraci, G. Duodenal and rectal mucosa inflammation in patients with non–celiac wheat sensitivity. *Clin. Gastroenterol. Hepatol.* **2019**, *17*, 682–690. [CrossRef]
61. Zanini, B.; Villanacci, V.; Marullo, M.; Cadei, M.; Lanzarotto, F.; Bozzola, A.; Ricci, C. Duodenal histological features in suspected non-celiac gluten sensitivity: New insights into a still undefined condition. *Virchows Arch.* **2018**, *473*, 229–234. [CrossRef]
62. Losurdo, G.; Piscitelli, D.; Pezzuto, F.; Fortarezza, F.; Covelli, C.; Marra, A.; Iannone, A.; Amoruso, A.; Principi, M.; Ierardi, E. T helper lymphocyte and mast cell immunohistochemical pattern in nonceliac gluten sensitivity. *Gastroenterol. Res. Pract.* **2017**, *2017*, 5023680. [CrossRef]
63. Losurdo, G.; Giorgio, F.; Piscitelli, D.; Montenegro, L.; Covelli, C.; Fiore, M.G.; Giangaspero, A.; Iannone, A.; Principi, M.; Amoruso, A. May the assessment of baseline mucosal molecular pattern predict the development of gluten related disorders among microscopic enteritis? *World J. Gastroenterol.* **2016**, *22*, 8017. [CrossRef]
64. Brottveit, M.; Beitnes, A.-C.R.; Tollefsen, S.; Bratlie, J.E.; Jahnsen, F.L.; Johansen, F.-E.; Sollid, L.M.; Lundin, K.E. Mucosal cytokine response after short-term gluten challenge in celiac disease and non-celiac gluten sensitivity. *Am. J. Gastroenterol.* **2013**, *108*, 842. [CrossRef]
65. Brottveit, M.; Ráki, M.; Bergseng, E.; Fallang, L.-E.; Simonsen, B.; Løvik, A.; Larsen, S.; Løberg, E.M.; Jahnsen, F.L.; Sollid, L.M. Assessing possible celiac disease by an HLA-DQ2-gliadin tetramer test. *Am. J. Gastroenterol.* **2011**, *106*, 1318. [CrossRef]
66. Ontiveros, N.; Tye-Din, J.; Hardy, M.; Anderson, R. Ex-vivo whole blood secretion of interferon (IFN)-γ and IFN-γ-inducible protein-10 measured by enzyme-linked immunosorbent assay are as sensitive as IFN-γ enzyme-linked immunospot for the detection of gluten-reactive T cells in human leucocyte antigen (HLA)-DQ 2·5+-associated coeliac disease. *Clin. Exp. Immunol.* **2014**, *175*, 305–315.

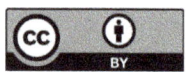

© 2019 by the authors. Licensee MDPI, Basel, Switzerland. This article is an open access article distributed under the terms and conditions of the Creative Commons Attribution (CC BY) license (http://creativecommons.org/licenses/by/4.0/).

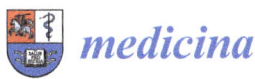

Review

Pediatric Celiac Disease in Central and East Asia: Current Knowledge and Prevalence

Dimitri Poddighe [1,*], Marzhan Rakhimzhanova [2], Yelena Marchenko [3] and Carlo Catassi [4]

1. Department of Medicine, Nazarbayev University School of Medicine, 010000 Astana, Kazakhstan
2. Department of Pediatrics, National Research Center of Mother and Child Health, University Medical Center, 010000 Astana, Kazakhstan; Marzhan.Rahimzhanova@umc.org.kz
3. Center of Laboratory Medicine, Republican Diagnostic Center, University Medical Center, 010000 Astana, Kazakhstan; elena.martchenko@gmail.com
4. Department of Pediatrics, Universita' Politecnica delle Marche, 60121 Ancona, Italy; c.catassi@univpm.it
* Correspondence: dimitri.poddighe@nu.edu.kz; Tel.: +7-7172-694637

Received: 12 December 2018; Accepted: 3 January 2019; Published: 12 January 2019

Abstract: The current prevalence of pediatric Celiac Disease (CD) is estimated to be around 1% in the general population, worldwide. However, according to the geographic area, a great variability of CD prevalence has been described. Whereas a number of studies are available from Europe, North and South America, Australia, South-West Asia, and North Africa, the knowledge and awareness of CD in large parts of the remaining world areas is definitively poor. In several countries of Central and East Asia, the consumption of wheat is consistent and/or has significantly increased in recent decades, and CD is supposed to be underdiagnosed in children. In this mini-review, we aimed to summarize the current knowledge about the prevalence of pediatric CD in Central and East Asia, paying attention to the HLA-DQ immunogenetic background as well. Indeed, CD is likely not to be as uncommon as previously or currently thought in countries like Russia, Kazakhstan, and China, in addition to India, where pediatric CD has been clearly showed to be quite prevalent. Therefore, there is an urgent need for population-based studies on the prevalence of CD in those countries, especially in children, in order to increase the awareness of this disease and to improve the diagnostic strategy in these areas.

Keywords: celiac disease; children; HLA-DQ; prevalence; Asia

1. Introduction

Celiac disease (CD) is a multifactorial immune-mediated disorder, triggered by the ingestion of gluten and other gluten-related proteins in genetically predisposed subjects. HLA-DQ alleles, coding α and β chains of MHC-DQ2 and -DQ8 heterodimers, have been shown to be a necessary—but not sufficient—immunogenetic background for the development of CD. Moreover, gluten is the required environmental exposure to develop CD in genetically predisposed individuals, probably in addition to other variable constitutional and/or acquired factors [1–3].

CD is a systemic disease, as the clinical manifestations are not limited to the intestinal tract: indeed, it is estimated that a significant portion of CD cases are currently undiagnosed, and its great clinical heterogeneity with 'atypical' and variable extra-intestinal manifestations is undoubtedly a major contributing factor [4,5]. However, the growing awareness about CD among patients and physicians has drawn specific attention on this diagnosis and even prompted a great debate on widened screening strategies in Western countries. Because of this, the actual and estimated prevalence rates of CD have increased significantly in the last few decades [6,7]. Even in some countries where CD was considered to be nonexistent or negligible until recent years, this disease has been found to be quite frequent and, in some populations, recent immunogenetic analyses and epidemiological data suggested that CD prevalence and risk may be comparable to Europe and North America [8].

Despite a wide variation in prevalence according to the geographic area, pediatric CD is currently considered to affect almost 1% of the general population worldwide. Indeed, CD is frequent in Europe, North and South America, Australia, South-West Asia, and North Africa, where more than 30% of the population carry the DQ2 haplotype and high consumption of wheat is present. In contrast, CD is extremely rare in Far East Asia and in sub-Saharan Africa, where wheat and other gluten cereals are not staple foods [9].

As mentioned above, during the last few years several studies have also suggested CD to be common in South West Asia. Population screening studies have been carried out in Iran, Turkey and Israel, where the prevalence figured comparable to Europe [10,11]. However, in most other parts of Asia, data on CD prevalence are scarce or even totally absent. As the consumption of wheat is actually consistent in several of these areas [12], a high number of unrecognized CD cases may actually exist, and be undiagnosed because of poor awareness of this disease.

In this mini-review, we aim to summarize the current knowledge about pediatric CD in Central and East Asia, where very few studies and research are currently available through the Medline/Pubmed database, except for the Indian subcontinent. The specific Asian areas that have been discussed in each section of this review are graphically represented in Figure 1. This article organization by geographical macro-areas will help readers to understand and appreciate the wide differences in the knowledge of pediatric CD epidemiology and disease awareness among countries of non-Western Asia, where many more studies on this topic have been carried out so far.

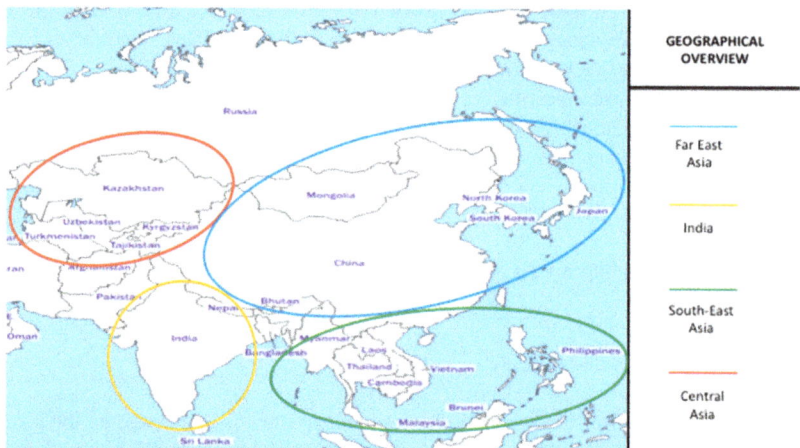

Figure 1. Overview of the geographical macro-areas of Central and East Asia, as discussed in each section of the review.

2. Far East Asia

In Japan, the overall prevalence of the HLA-DQ2 and -DQ8 immunotypes has been reported to be quite low, according to a study including 371 unrelated healthy apheresis blood donors assessed by high-resolution HLA typing. In detail, whereas the allele frequency of the HLA-DQB1*02 allele was 0.3%, the frequency of DQB1*03:02 allele was actually 10.8% [13].

In addition to such a low prevalence of HLA-DQ genotypes leading to susceptibility for CD, the dietary intake of wheat in Japan is still one-third of what is observed in Western countries, although the consumption of these products has been increasing in last few years [14]. However, a very recent study by Fukunaga et al. confirmed that CD is still of low prevalence in the Japanese population, as this diagnosis was confirmed in only 0.05% of 2008 asymptomatic people having their annual check-up [15]. Unfortunately, no study is currently available about CD prevalence in Japanese children.

As for China, CD is not so rare as previously thought. Recently, Kou et al. found a prevalence of 2.85% in 246 adult patients referred for irritable bowel syndrome [16]. In this same clinical setting, another study from South China observed a 1.01% prevalence; interestingly, CD was diagnosed in 0.28% of the controls [17]. However, the meta-analysis by Juan et al. is the best source of genetic data about CD predisposition in China so far. According to this paper, published in 2013, the pooled frequencies of the DQA1*05-DQB1*02 (MHC-DQ2 genotype) and DQA1*03-DQB1*03:02 (MHC-DQ8 genotype) alleles were 3.40% and 2.10%, respectively. However, the frequency of the DQB1* 02:01 allele was as much as 10.5% overall; importantly, among all Chinese regions where the pooled data came from, significant variations were observed (from 22.04% in Xinjiang Uygur region to 2.8% in Yunnan province). Basically, this allele was more common in northern China than in the southern Chinese populations [18]. More recently, the same group reported positivity for CD serum markers in 2.19% of almost 20,000 Chinese adolescents and young students (16–25 years), who underwent routine physical examinations in two universities. However, most of them tested positive for anti-DGP IgG, whereas only 0.36% were positive for anti-tTG IgA; moreover, no information was provided about the histopathological findings of duodenal biopsy, if performed [19]. There are some other studies from China reporting anti-tTG IgA serology in Chinese patients affected with diabetes mellitus type I (DMT1) and autoimmune thyroid diseases, who were positive in 22% of cases, globally [20]. However, other than that, the only available study on pediatric CD in China described 14 patients diagnosed with CD after screening 118 children affected with chronic diarrhea. Here, CD was found in 11.9% of the study cohort and all children (1–12 years) underwent duodenal mucosal biopsy, after the detection of anti-tTG IgA ($n = 14$) and EMA ($n = 9$) positivity [21].

Unfortunately, no informative articles were retrieved from Korean peninsula and Mongolia about pediatric CD.

3. India

In 2002, Kaur et al. provided the first study assessing the HLA background in pediatric CD patients from India. They investigated 117 children with gastrointestinal (e.g., chronic diarrhea, abdominal pain) and extra-gastrointestinal (short stature, iron-deficient anemia, failure to thrive, etc.) manifestations who received a diagnosis of CD by intestinal biopsy: importantly, almost 100% association with DQB1*02:01 in these Indian pediatric CD patients was reported [22]. In general, according to the study by Ramakrishna et al., the prevalence of genes determining MHC-DQ2 and/or -DQ8 expression in the Indian population was around 35%; moreover, the disease prevalence was estimated to be around 1%. CD diagnosis was more frequent in the northern part of India, where the mean daily wheat intake is the highest [11].

Interestingly, an American study of nearly 500,000 duodenal biopsy samples (from all over the USA) showed that the ethnic group from the Punjab area (northern India) had the greatest prevalence of villous atrophy among all the ethnicities living in the country (3.08% vs. 1.80% for other Americans) [23]. Accordingly, in a cross sectional study involving urban and rural populations ($n = 10,488$) in the northern part of India, the overall serological prevalence of CD was 1.44%, and the overall prevalence of CD was 1.04% [24]. Moreover, Agrawal et al. provided detailed HLA immunogenetic data from 1336 unrelated healthy people from northern and northeastern India. As regards MHC-DQ2 and MHC-DQ8 alleles, these authors provided the following frequencies (highest–lowest), variable according to the region: DQA1*05:01 (11.20–16.70%), DQB1*02:01 (17.40–26.50%), DQA1*03:01 (9.50–24.10%) and DQB1*03:02 (0–5.48%) [25].

As regards the pediatric population in India, despite these findings, Sood et al. reported 0.3–0.4% CD prevalence in Punjab children and adolescents (3–17 years). However, this prevalence may have been under-estimated, as only selected groups of children were screened, based upon a structured questionnaire; thus, only these patients received a full medical assessment, including CD serology.

At that time, this publication was the first large-scale study on pediatric CD (including 4347 children undergone serologic screening): it demonstrated that pediatric CD in India was more common than previously appreciated, especially in wheat-eating parts of India [26]. Conversely, Batthacharya et al. reported around 1% CD prevalence in 400 consecutive children (1–12 years) undergoing venipuncture for any reason, who were referred to the general pediatric department of a tertiary care hospital of Northern India [27]. Moreover, Srivastava et al. showed that the prevalence of CD diagnosed in the first-degree relatives (FDRs) of CD children from Northern India was 4.4%, 14 times higher than in the general population [28]. In particular, as concerns the pediatric FDRs of children diagnosed with CD, Singla et al. reported 9-fold higher CD prevalence than in the general pediatric population, with peaks in symptomatic FDRs affected with anemia and short stature [29]. Previously, Gautam et al. had investigated 63 siblings (2–15 years) of 48 CD children, and 22% were shown to have CD as well. Importantly, two third of them did not report any gastrointestinal symptoms suggestive of CD [30].

On the contrary, in Southern India CD is less frequent, which has been related to the effect of both genetic and environmental factors. Indeed, Yachha et al. highlighted that the frequency of celiac HLA-DQ predisposing alleles was much higher in Northern India (31.9%) than in Southern India (9–12.8%), where this genetic difference is coupled with a different staple diet based upon rice dishes [31].

4. South-East Asia

In most countries of South-East Asia, the frequency of HLA-DQB1*02 is estimated to be between 5–20% [14].

In Vietnam, CD is considered a very rare disease, although the frequency of MHC-DQ2/DQ8 alleles is not particularly low. The scarce exposure to gluten is supposed to be responsible for this epidemiological situation. Zanella et al. investigated the celiac autoimmunity in 1961 Vietnamese children having blood drawn for any reason. Around 1% of these children (median age: 5.3 years) were positive for anti-tTG IgA; however, among them, only 33% resulted to be carriers of any MHC-DQ2/DQ8 alleles, and no duodenal histopathological data were provided in this study [32].

In Thailand, Thammarakcharoen et al. assessed the frequency of HLA-DQB1*02 and DQB1*03:02 alleles, in addition to anti-tTG serology, in children with DMT1. HLA-DQB1*02 and HLA-DQB1*03:02 allele frequencies were 27% and 14% in DMT1 patients and normal controls, respectively. Only one patient was positive for anti-tTG IgA, and he was asymptomatic [33]. Therefore, the prevalence of CD screening positivity seems to be currently negligible in Thai children.

No pediatric studies were retrieved from Malaysia. However, Yap et al. reported unexpectedly high seroprevalence of CD autoantibodies (1.25%) in healthy young adults from the Malaysian population. Importantly, Malaysia has a multiracial population consisting of three major ethnic groups (Malay, Chinese, and Indian), which may affect the genetic predisposition to CD. Unfortunately, HLA haplotyping was not performed in this study and intestinal histological data were not provided [34].

Finally, no relevant studies about pediatric CD were retrieved from other countries of South-East Asia (Laos, Myanmar, Bangladesh, Singapore, Indonesia, Philippines).

5. Central Asia

Clinical data about the prevalence of CD in the countries of Central Asia (Kazakhstan, Kyrgyzstan, Tajikistan, Turkmenistan, and Uzbekistan) from English-language medical literature are extremely scarce.

However, a paper by Savvateeva et al. first provided an overview on CD in Russia and, interestingly, also cited some references of studies coming from the surrounding republics of Central Asia [35]. Therefore, some more information about CD in Central Asia could be obtained from Russian-language medical sources. Importantly, as for Russia specifically, most studies considered in the aforementioned article included children and, according to these authors, the estimation of pediatric CD prevalence in this country has increased from about 0.02% to 0.3% during the first decade of 2000s. Moreover, in children with consistent clinical manifestations and/or specific risk factors (e.g., autoimmune diseases, Down syndrome, etc.), CD prevalence proved to be comparable to Europe (0.94% to 15.98%, according to the specific clinical setting). Additionally, Savvateeva et al. reported data on the polymorphic variants of HLA-DQA1 and -DQB1 genes in CD patients from the cities of Tomsk and Krasnodar (which are located in Russia, north and west of Kazakhstan respectively) and from Yakutia (Eastern Russia). These studies (all published in Russian) suggested that the allelic frequencies of CD-related HLA-DQ genes in those populations may be comparable to those observed in Europe [35].

We traced back some of the primary sources describing those data, which were published in Russian-written journals. The study by Kurtanov et al. examined 37 children (1–18 years) affected with gastrointestinal symptoms; here, an interesting finding was a relative abundance of CD patients carrying the MHC-DQ8 genotype, which was found in > 30% of Yakuts patients [36]. Tlif et al. authored a study from Krasnodar which included 110 children with DMT1 and 654 controls, whereby the respective frequencies of CD predisposing HLA-DQ alleles were as follows: DQA1*05:01 (28.6% and 29%), DQB1*02:01 (33.6% and 19.5%), DQA1*03:01 (38.2% and 12.2%), and DQB1*03:02 (31.6% and 8.3%). Among these DMT1 patients, 32 children were diagnosed with CD and they showed the following genotype distribution: DQA1*05:01 (40.6%), DQB1*0201 (35.9%), DQA1* 03:01 (9.4%), and DQB1*03:02 (7.8%). Therefore, this study showed a relative proportion between MHC-DQ2 and MHC-DQ8 alleles that seems to follow the same trend described in Europe [37].

The only study from Kazakhstan (again, cited by Savvateeva et al.) was authored in Russian language by Sharipova: this author described patients from the Almaty region, which is located in the southern part of the country. Starting from 17,800 pediatric patients registered in two clinics of the city, this author considered 6,380 children who displayed gastrointestinal symptoms and/or malnutrition, or had autoimmune diseases (such as thyroiditis and DMT1) or a sibling affected with CD. Among them, the author selected a group of 1,220 children as 'at risk for CD' based on the clinical examination; however, no precise inclusion criteria were described. One out of three children were then randomly chosen to undergo assessment of antigliadin antibodies (AGA) IgG and IgA titers, meaning that around 400 children received this screening. Finally, 86 children were positive to AGA IgA and/or IgG, and 74 of them (aged 3–15 years) were reported as affected with CD according to their histopathological results (however, once again, no detailed description was provided). Based on this study, the CD detection rate was 1 case in every 18 screened children, which allowed this author to estimate a CD prevalence of 1:262 children in Kazakhstan [38]. It is evident that such an experimental approach had several limitations, as selection and analysis bias may have been introduced in this numerical estimation, in addition to the poorly sensitive and specific screening protocol. Indeed, very recently Verma et al. confirmed that almost 40% of anti-tTG IgA positive celiac children are missed when using a screening approach based on AGA IgA only [39].

Moreover, this study from Kazakhstan also reported the genetic analysis of MHC-DQ2 and MHC-DQ8 related alleles: these results were not displayed in detail, but it is very interesting to notice that the frequency of these susceptibility alleles in CD children was apparently approximately 60% only [38]. Actually, this finding might raise some further concerns about the diagnosis of CD, considering the very high, almost absolute, negative predictive value associated with the complete absence of any of the alleles coding α and β chains of MHC-DQ2 and -DQ8 heterodimers [3]. However, even CD children included in the available studies from Central and Eastern Russia were shown to carry these alleles with a significantly lower frequency than expected, namely around 80% [35].

As regards other countries of Central Asia, even the research in the Russian literature was scant. However, Abduzhabarova et al. published an article in English providing some data about the HLA immunogenetic profile in 54 Uzbek children (aged 1–14 years) diagnosed with CD. Although it was not possible to retrieve the raw data, 36 CD children (around 70%) were shown to carry MHC-DQ2 alleles, but data related MHC-DQ8 alleles were not available. However, an interesting point is that around 36% of their 109 healthy control children were carriers of MHC-DQ2 alleles, which is consistent with prevalence data observed in the European general population [40].

6. Conclusions

Except for Indian children, epidemiological studies and clinical research about pediatric CD from Central and East Asia are lacking or poor. However, there is initial evidence that the MHC-DQ2 and MHC-DQ8 immunogenetic background is not so unusual in several populations from these areas as previously or commonly thought. Indeed, in South-East Asia the frequency of HLA-DQB1*02 is estimated to be comprised between 5–20%, and in Central Asia the prevalence of HLA-DQ alleles predisposing to CD may be even higher. As concerns the disease occurrence, the exposure to the environmental trigger, namely gluten, currently makes the difference among different countries in Asia. Whereas in Vietnam and Thailand the CD prevalence is still negligible because of the rice-based dietary regimen, in Russia and in the Republics of Central Asia the occurrence of CD seems to be growing, given the large consumption of wheat. Indeed, the wheat consumption per person per year is estimated to be lower than 25–50 kg in most regions of South-East Asia, whereas it does exceed 150 kg in Kazakhstan, Uzbekistan, Tajikistan, Kyrgyzstan, and Turkmenistan [12].

However, such a CD epidemiological burden has not been clearly evidenced yet, probably because the disease is actively sought only in the presence of (severe) gastrointestinal manifestations, and the access to CD diagnostic procedures is still limited for several reasons. Therefore, it is essential to implement cost-effective diagnostic protocols that can allow the rest of the 'celiac iceberg' to emerge, considering the potential and persistent health consequences related to the under-diagnosis of CD in children. Indeed, this under-diagnosis may also represent an important issue of public health, especially in those countries where the birth rate is significantly higher and the population is relatively younger than in Western countries.

In conclusion, it is likely that CD is not so uncommon, even in several Asian countries other than India and Western Asia. Therefore, there is urgent need for population-based studies on the prevalence of CD in these countries, especially in Russia and Central Asia, in order to increase the awareness of this disease and to improve the diagnostic strategy.

Author Contributions: D.P. conceived and wrote the paper. M.R. and Y.M. contributed in the literature research, including the manuscript in Russian language. C.C. provided important intellectual contributions.

Funding: This research received no external funding.

Conflicts of Interest: The authors declare no conflict of interest. Carlo Catassi has served as scientific consultant for Schaer, Burgstall (BZ), Italy and NOOS S.r.l., Rome, Italy.

References

1. Di Sabatino, A.; Corazza, G.R. Coeliac disease. *Lancet* **2009**, *373*, 1480–1493. [CrossRef]
2. Lionetti, E.; Castellaneta, S.; Francavilla, R.; Pulvirenti, A.; Tonutti, E.; Amarri, S.; Barbato, M.; Barbera, C.; Barera, G.; Bellantoni, A.; et al. Introduction of gluten, HLA status, and the risk of celiac disease in children. *N. Engl. J. Med.* **2014**, *371*, 1295–1303. [CrossRef] [PubMed]
3. De Silvestri, A.; Capittini, C.; Poddighe, D.; Valsecchi, C.; Marseglia, G.L.; Tagliacarne, S.C.; Scotti, V.; Rebuffi, C.; Pasi, A.; Martinetti, M.; et al. HLA-DQ genetics in children with celiac disease: A meta-analysis suggesting a two-step genetic screening procedure starting with HLA-DQ β chains. *Pediatr. Res.* **2018**, *83*, 564–572. [CrossRef] [PubMed]
4. Husby, S.; Koletzko, S.; Korponay-Szabó, I.R.; Mearin, M.L.; Phillips, A.; Shamir, R.; Troncone, R.; ESPGHAN Working Group on Coeliac Disease Diagnosis; ESPGHAN Gastroenterology Committee; European Society for Pediatric Gastroenterology, Hepatology, and Nutrition; et al. European Society for Pediatric Gastroenterology, Hepatology, and Nutrition guidelines for the diagnosis of coeliac disease. *J. Pediatr. Gastroenterol. Nutr.* **2012**, *54*, 136–160. [CrossRef] [PubMed]

5. Admou, B.; Essaadouni, L.; Krati, K.; Zaher, K.; Sbihi, M.; Chabaa, L.; Belaabidia, B.; Alaoui-Yazidi, A. Atypical celiac disease: From recognizing to managing. *Gastroenterol. Res. Pract.* **2012**, *2012*, 637187. [CrossRef] [PubMed]
6. Wessels, M.M.S.; de Rooij, N.; Roovers, L.; Verhage, J.; de Vries, W.; Mearin, M.L. Towards an individual screening strategy for first-degree relatives of celiac patients. *Eur. J. Pediatr.* **2018**, *177*, 1585–1592. [CrossRef] [PubMed]
7. Poddighe, D. Individual screening strategy for pediatric celiac disease. *Eur. J. Pediatr.* **2018**, *177*, 1871. [CrossRef]
8. Singh, P.; Arora, A.; Strand, T.A.; Leffler, D.A.; Catassi, C.; Green, P.H.; Kelly, C.P.; Ahuja, V.; Makharia, G.K. Global Prevalence of Celiac Disease: Systematic Review and Meta-analysis. *Clin. Gastroenterol. Hepatol.* **2018**, *16*, 823–836. [CrossRef]
9. Catassi, C.; Gatti, S.; Lionetti, E. World perspective and celiac disease epidemiology. *Dig. Dis.* **2015**, *33*, 141–146. [CrossRef]
10. Singh, P.; Arora, S.; Singh, A.; Strand, T.A.; Makharia, G.K. Prevalence of celiac disease in Asia: A systematic review and meta-analysis. *J. Gastroenterol. Hepatol.* **2016**, *31*, 1095–1101. [CrossRef]
11. Ramakrishna, B.S.; Makharia, G.K.; Chetri, K.; Dutta, S.; Mathur, P.; Ahuja, V.; Amarchand, R.; Balamurugan, R.; Chowdhury, S.D.; Daniel, D.; et al. Prevalence of Adult Celiac Disease in India: Regional Variations and Associations. *Am. J. Gastroenterol.* **2016**, *111*, 115–123. [CrossRef] [PubMed]
12. Rostami Nejad, M.; Rostami, K.; Emami, M.; Zali, M.; Malekzadeh, R. Epidemiology of celiac disease in iran: A review. *Middle East J. Dig. Dis.* **2011**, *3*, 5–12. [PubMed]
13. Saito, S.; Ota, S.; Yamada, E.; Inoko, H.; Ota, M. Allele frequencies and haplotypic associations defined by allelic DNA typing at HLA class I and class II loci in the Japanese population. *Tissue Antigens* **2000**, *56*, 522–529. [CrossRef] [PubMed]
14. Cummins, A.G.; Roberts-Thomson, I.C. Prevalence of celiac disease in the Asia-Pacific region. *J. Gastroenterol. Hepatol.* **2009**, *24*, 1347–1351. [CrossRef] [PubMed]
15. Fukunaga, M.; Ishimura, N.; Fukuyama, C.; Izumi, D.; Ishikawa, N.; Araki, A.; Oka, A.; Mishiro, T.; Ishihara, S.; Maruyama, R.; et al. Celiac disease in non-clinical populations of Japan. *J. Gastroenterol.* **2018**, *53*, 208–214. [CrossRef] [PubMed]
16. Kou, G.J.; Guo, J.; Zuo, X.L.; Li, C.Q.; Liu, C.; Ji, R.; Liu, H.; Wang, X.; Li, Y.Q. Prevalence of celiac disease in adult Chinese patients with diarrhea-predominant irritable bowel syndrome: A prospective, controlled, cohort study. *J. Dig. Dis.* **2018**, *19*, 136–143. [CrossRef] [PubMed]
17. Wang, H.; Zhou, G.; Luo, L.; Crusius, J.B.; Yuan, A.; Kou, J.; Yang, G.; Wang, M.; Wu, J.; von Blomberg, B.M.; et al. Serological Screening for Celiac Disease in Adult Chinese Patients With Diarrhea Predominant Irritable Bowel Syndrome. *Medicine* **2015**, *94*, e1779. [CrossRef] [PubMed]
18. Yuan, J.; Gao, J.; Li, X.; Liu, F.; Wijmenga, C.; Chen, H.; Gilissen, L.J. The tip of the "celiac iceberg" in China: A systematic review and meta-analysis. *PLoS ONE* **2013**, *8*, e81151. [CrossRef]
19. Yuan, J.; Zhou, C.; Gao, J.; Li, J.; Yu, F.; Lu, J.; Li, X.; Wang, X.; Tong, P.; Wu, Z.; et al. Prevalence of Celiac Disease Autoimmunity Among Adolescents and Young Adults in China. *Clin. Gastroenterol. Hepatol.* **2017**, *15*, 1572–1579. [CrossRef]
20. Zhao, Z.; Zou, J.; Zhao, L.; Cheng, Y.; Cai, H.; Li, M.; Liu, E.; Yu, L.; Liu, Y. Celiac Disease Autoimmunity in Patients with Autoimmune Diabetes and Thyroid Disease among Chinese Population. *PLoS ONE* **2016**, *11*, e0157510. [CrossRef]
21. Wang, X.Q.; Liu, W.; Xu, C.D.; Mei, H.; Gao, Y.; Peng, H.M.; Yuan, L.; Xu, J.J. Celiac disease in children with diarrhea in 4 cities in China. *J. Pediatr. Gastroenterol. Nutr.* **2011**, *53*, 368–370. [PubMed]
22. Kaur, G.; Sarkar, N.; Bhatnagar, S.; Kumar, S.; Rapthap, C.C.; Bhan, M.K.; Mehra, N.K. Pediatric celiac disease in India is associated with multiple DR3-DQ2 haplotypes. *Hum. Immunol.* **2002**, *63*, 677–682. [CrossRef]
23. Krigel, A.; Turner, K.O.; Makharia, G.K.; Green, P.H.; Genta, R.M.; Lebwohl, B. Ethnic Variations in Duodenal Villous Atrophy Consistent with Celiac Disease in the United States. *Clin. Gastroenterol. Hepatol.* **2016**, *14*, 1105–1111. [CrossRef]
24. Makharia, G.K.; Verma, A.K.; Amarchand, R.; Bhatnagar, S.; Das, P.; Goswami, A.; Bhatia, V.; Ahuja, V.; Datta Gupta, S.; Anand, K. Prevalence of celiac disease in the northern part of India: A community based study. *J. Gastroenterol. Hepatol.* **2011**, *26*, 894–900. [CrossRef]

25. Agrawal, S.; Srivastava, S.K.; Borkar, M.; Chaudhuri, T.K. Genetic affinities of north and northeastern populations of India: Inference from HLA-based study. *Tissue Antigens* **2008**, *72*, 120–130. [CrossRef] [PubMed]
26. Sood, A.; Midha, V.; Sood, N.; Avasthi, G.; Sehgal, A. Prevalence of celiac disease among school children in Punjab, North India. *J. Gastroenterol. Hepatol.* **2006**, *21*, 1622–1625. [CrossRef] [PubMed]
27. Bhattacharya, M.; Dubey, A.P.; Mathur, N.B. Prevalence of celiac disease in north Indian children. *Indian Pediatr.* **2009**, *46*, 415–417.
28. Srivastava, A.; Yachha, S.K.; Mathias, A.; Parveen, F.; Poddar, U.; Agrawal, S. Prevalence, human leukocyte antigen typing and strategy for screening among Asian first-degree relatives of children with celiac disease. *J. Gastroenterol. Hepatol.* **2010**, *25*, 319–324. [CrossRef]
29. Singla, S.; Kumar, P.; Singh, P.; Kaur, G.; Rohtagi, A.; Choudhury, M. HLA Profile of Celiac Disease among First-Degree Relatives from a Tertiary Care Center in North India. *Indian J. Pediatr.* **2016**, *83*, 1248–1252. [CrossRef]
30. Gautam, A.; Jain, B.K.; Midha, V.; Sood, A.; Sood, N. Prevalence of celiac disease among siblings of celiac disease patients. *Indian J. Gastroenterol.* **2006**, *25*, 233–235.
31. Yachha, S.K.; Poddar, U. Celiac disease in India. *Indian J. Gastroenterol.* **2007**, *26*, 230–237. [PubMed]
32. Zanella, S.; De Leo, L.; Nguyen-Ngoc-Quynh, L.; Nguyen-Duy, B.; Not, T.; Tran-Thi-Chi, M.; Phung-Duc, S.; Le-Thanh, H.; Malaventura, C.; Vatta, S.; et al. Cross-sectional study of coeliac autoimmunity in a population of Vietnamese children. *BMJ Open* **2016**, *6*, e011173. [CrossRef] [PubMed]
33. Thammarakcharoen, T.; Hirankarn, N.; Sahakitrungruang, T.; Thongmee, T.; Kuptawintu, P.; Kanoonthong, S.; Chongsrisawat, V. Frequency of HLA-DQB1*0201/02 and DQB1*0302 alleles and tissue transglutaminase antibody seropositivity in children with type 1 diabetes mellitus. *Asian Pac. J. Allergy Immunol.* **2017**, *35*, 82–85. [PubMed]
34. Yap, T.W.; Chan, W.K.; Leow, A.H.; Azmi, A.N.; Loke, M.F.; Vadivelu, J.; Goh, K.L. Prevalence of serum celiac antibodies in a multiracial Asian population-a first study in the young Asian adult population of Malaysia. *PLoS ONE* **2015**, *10*, e0121908. [CrossRef] [PubMed]
35. Savvateeva, L.V.; Erdes, S.I.; Antishin, A.S.; Zamyatnin, A.A., Jr. Overview of Celiac Disease in Russia: Regional Data and Estimated Prevalence. *J. Immunol. Res.* **2017**, *2017*, 2314813. [CrossRef] [PubMed]
36. Kurtanov, H.A.; Danilova, A.L.; Yakovleva, A.E.; Savvina, A.D.; Maximova, H.P. Genetic research of HLA genes I and II class—DRB1, DQA1, DQB1 in patients with celiac disease. *Bull. Hematol.* **2015**, *11*, 44–47. (In Russian)
37. Tlif, A.I.; Kondratyeva, E.I.; Chernyak, I.Y.; Dolbneva, O.V.; Shtoda, I.I.; Golovenko, I.M. The prevalence of polymorphisms of genes HLA DQA1 and DQB1 in patients with type 1 diabetes and celiac disease in the Krasnodar Region. *Kuban Sci. Med. Bull.* **2012**, *5*, 65–69. (In Russian)
38. Sharipova, M.N. Clinical, epidemiological and genetic characteristics of celiac disease in children in Kazakhstan. *Pediatr. Named G.N. Speransky* **2009**, *87*, 106–108. (In Russian)
39. Verma, A.K.; Gatti, S.; Lionetti, E.; Galeazzi, T.; Monachesi, C.; Franceschini, E.; Balanzoni, L.; Scattolo, N.; Cinquetti, M.; Catassi, C. Comparison of Diagnostic Performance of the IgA Anti-tTG Test vs IgA Anti-Native Gliadin Antibodies Test in Detection of Celiac Disease in the General Population. *Clin. Gastroenterol. Hepatol.* **2018**, *16*, 1997–1998. [CrossRef]
40. Abduzhabarova, Z.M. Immunogenetic Profile in children with celiac disease from Uzbek population. *Eur. Sci. Rev.* **2016**, *3–4*, 34–36. [CrossRef]

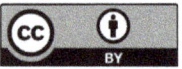

© 2019 by the authors. Licensee MDPI, Basel, Switzerland. This article is an open access article distributed under the terms and conditions of the Creative Commons Attribution (CC BY) license (http://creativecommons.org/licenses/by/4.0/).

MDPI
St. Alban-Anlage 66
4052 Basel
Switzerland
Tel. +41 61 683 77 34
Fax +41 61 302 89 18
www.mdpi.com

Medicina Editorial Office
E-mail: medicina@mdpi.com
www.mdpi.com/journal/medicina

www.ingramcontent.com/pod-product-compliance
Lightning Source LLC
LaVergne TN
LVHW070553100526
838202LV00012B/454